EAT

LESS PLASTIC

DRINK

MORE ROCKS

COMMON SENSE HEALTH

TIPS FOR AN INSANE WORLD

FIRST PUBLISHED AND PRINTED IN THE UNITED KINGDOM 2003

BY REGENERATION PUBLISHING
AISLABY, NORTH YORKSHIRE. YO18 8PE

ISBN   0 – 9543281 – 0 – 8

The information contained in this book is for educational purposes only. The Author, Publisher and Retailer accept no liability for damages arising out of the abuse of the information contained herein. In addition, the information in this book is not intended to replace the advice of an appropriate healthcare professional.

ACKNOWLEDGEMENTS

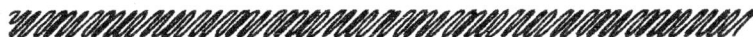

My sincere thanks go to:

Karin Doose for typing beyond the call of duty.

Charlotte Hamlyn and Shelly Cawood for typesetting and graphics that turned a mountain of pages into something that looks like a real book.

Alan Rudgard for creating the final product.

Finally, my love to my wife Stacey, my daughter Kyla and my two boys, Ansel and Seren, for their belief, help and support through difficult times.

CONTENTS

THE BEGINNING

In 1983, I cured myself of the bone disease osteomyelitis using dietary changes combined with simple treatments from oriental folk medicine.

I had suffered from this painful and debilitating condition for 16 years so, as you can imagine, I was more than pleased with my recovery. As the weeks progressed, I was able to bear more weight on the affected leg than before and I was soon walking distances I hadn't thought possible for 16 years. I have had no recurrence of osteomyelitis since and, today, I live a fully active life with my family in North Yorkshire.

Friends encouraged me to tell my story. I made a number of media appearances and my recovery was featured in various newspapers and magazines. On a radio 'phone-in show, three consecutive calls revealed a very disturbing pattern in the treatment of the condition I'd had: the first was from a retired lady who, as a nurse between the wars, saw osteomyelitis effectively treated with clay plasters, good diet and bed rest (a similar approach to the one I'd employed); the second call was from a man my own age who'd had osteomyelitis in his foot. Surgeons had removed the bones from his foot so that he now had "a foot like a flipper". The osteomyelitis had, of course, simply appeared again further up his leg. His comment was: "What are they going to do now, chase it up my body, slashing as they go?" The final call was from a woman whose 8-year-old daughter had just been diagnosed with osteomyelitis in her ankle. The only option offered by the hospital was amputation of the girl's foot.

So, in a relatively short space of time, treatment for osteomyelitis had escalated from natural plasters to surgery and drugs, removal of bone (or replacement of it with steel or plastic, as had been planned in my case), and, finally, amputation.

Even with the experience I'd had, it still took me a few years to realise that highly inappropriate treatments were being applied in many other areas of modern medicine.

I went on to train in traditional systems of nutritional and preventive healthcare and, today, I give health and lifestyle advice here in the U.K. and abroad to individuals and groups. My approach is always the same: to show people how to regain control of their health and life direction.

The purpose of this book is to reach as many people as possible with this message, so that we can begin to reverse the growth of degenerative illness which has wrecked individual lives and devastated so many families in recent decades. The good news is that the truth about health is simpler than we are led to believe: cancer, heart disease and the rest are not inevitable.

Who is responsible for your health? The Prime Minister? The Pope? The overworked GP down the road? Once this truly sinks in, the way ahead is clear.

Make use of all the information and resources in this book to have your life work the way you want it to.

INTRODUCTION

We live in a world of illusion. Where our health is concerned, huge amounts of time, money and effort are put into modern medicine, yet we know the causes of most health problems (including the most serious) and choose to do nothing to prevent them. The idea that there are mysterious causes of illness which science is striving to discover is the greatest illusion of all - medical science is locked in battle with the *symptoms* of illness because that is where the money and glittering careers are to be had. If everybody got better, they'd be out of a job. Put another way, their jobs depend on people not getting better.

The major cause of death in the modern western world is heart disease. Second major cause is cancer. The third major cause of death is now, officially, western medicine which kills people with its inappropriate treatments (see 'Sack the Quack'). If you take into account the fact that doctors have known the causes of cancer and heart disease and how to prevent them for many years now, and have chosen to withhold the information in favour of expensive chemical and surgical treatments, this puts modern medicine right up to the top of the list as the major killer in the world today.

Don't get me wrong: I'm not denying that there are well-intentioned, hardworking and committed people in the medical industry. However, this book makes a heartfelt appeal for a wider approach to healthcare which encompasses prevention, the patient's own rôle in their recovery and safer treatments which are more effective in the long term than the quick-fix/miracle-cure, worry-about-the-problems-tomorrow approach of the profit-motivated drugs companies.

This book gives you the information that doctors don't tell you. Every chapter gives you clear and simple advice that will make a real difference to your health.

All that is required is to wake up to the fact that **no-one can take responsibility for your health but you**. Unless you take this responsibility, the only future you will have is one of *managed sickness* with someone else calling the shots at every turn.

I don't write books based upon statistics (which, as we all know, can be manipulated to prove or disprove anything.) I also don't promote clever theories (which invariably turn out to be inadequate or plain wrong a few years down the line.) The information here is based upon commonsense principles (which we abandon at our peril) handed down for countless centuries. The advice in this book is also based, most importantly, on the everyday experience of ordinary people, collected from advice sessions and educational workshops over the last 12 years (thanks, folks, your suffering has not been in vain!)

I don't know about you but, if I'm looking for information, I don't want to have to plough through 6 volumes of The Thoughts of Chairman John to get it. I want it fast and simple and very much to the point. That's the style of this book.

Read on.

NUTRITION

EAT LESS PLASTIC

"But I don't eat plastic!" I hear you cry. No? Well, there are numerous varieties of margarine and 'low fat spread', for example, which are so processed that, on the molecular level, they are closer to plastic than food. What are the long-term consequences of eating substances which the body can't even recognise as food?

Try an experiment. Buy one of these cheap, low fat spreads (the kind which contain no butter or dairy fats), leave it on the kitchen windowsill and forget about it. After a month or so, take a look: with many brands, nothing will have happened. Keep taking a look every few months: nothing wants to eat it! Insects, bacteria, nothing is interested - and neither should you be.

The best way to take oils and fats in the diet (aside from what is in natural food already) is to cook with extra virgin olive oil, sesame oil or similar cold-pressed organic oils from dark glass bottles. (Plastic and oil react to create substances which adversely affect the hormonal balance within the body, so plastic bottles are not a good idea unless you've got a sex-change in mind.)

While we're on the subject of plastic itself, avoid foods which are packed in plastic: the toxic qualities of the plastic leach into the food, resulting in the gender-bending effects (and others) mentioned above (see 'Don't Be A Woman".)

If you feel the need for oily spreads for bread,

crackers etc., then use natural quality peanut butter or tahini (sesame seed butter) kept in the fridge or other cool place so it doesn't become rancid. If your health is good, a little organic dairy butter now and again is OK. (Try making your own 'olive butter': mix half and half softened butter and olive oil. Keeps well in the fridge.)

If, for any reason you are unable to obtain good quality oils (for example, when travelling), take an Essential Fatty Acids supplement (for details of suppliers, contact the information line number at the end of this book.)

There's little chance of sustaining your health with highly processed substances. One of the biggest challenges to public health is that **people mistake products for food**. By the time your freezer-to-microwave TV dinner has found its way to your plate, it is so denatured and nutritionally inadequate you'd be as well off eating the cardboard box it came in.

We could go on to look at the use of petrochemical by-products in foods and medicines, 'natural flavourings' which are legally allowed to be 'nature identical flavourings' (i.e. totally synthetic) and many more, but I guess you're getting the idea by now.

The only way out of this nightmare will be to reinstate fresh foods and home cooking (see 'Buy Old Food') and to boost your depleted systems with minerals (see 'Drink More Rocks'.)

Oh, and one final highly technical tip as you navigate your way through the chemicals-masquerading-as-food minefield:

IF YOU CAN'T READ IT, DON'T EAT IT!

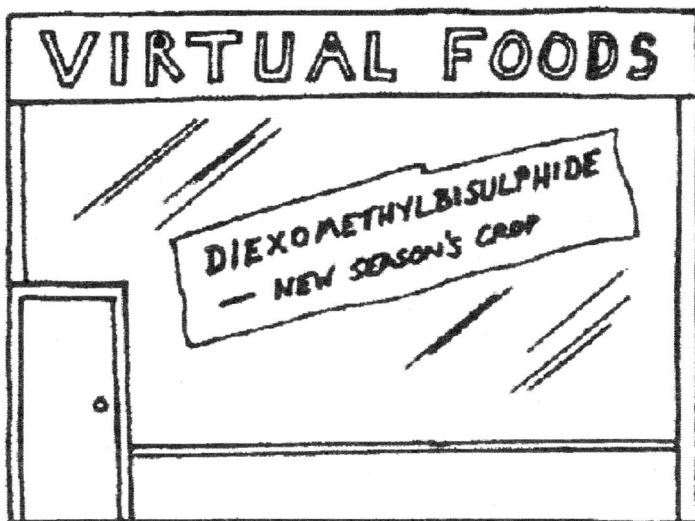

DRINK MORE ROCKS

If you're living in a remote countryside location, able to organically cultivate all of your own food on land which hasn't been farmed in the past 200 years, dressing the soil with mineral-rich seaweeds and rock dust, then don't read this.

Still with me? OK, here we go.

Of the 90 or so nutriments identified as being essential for human health, vitamins get the publicity every time (you'll tell me with confidence to eat oranges for vitamin C but where do I get rubidium?) Yet 67 of the 90 nutriments we need are minerals.

The insane practices of modern agribusiness have depleted the mineral content of our soil to levels never known before. Intensive farming has taken the 67 minerals out of the soil in the food which has been harvested from it. Farmers replace just three minerals - potassium, nitrogen and phosphorous - that leaves 64 to find.

As far back as 1936, a document was presented to the US Senate which stated quite plainly that there were no longer sufficient minerals in the soil to sustain human health - 70 years ago! So fundamental are minerals to our health, shortage of them is linked to a huge range of problems from osteoporosis to mental illness (see 'Beat the Sugar Blues'.)[1]

So, what to do?

Well, firstly increase the quality of your daily food, emphasizing fresh, local, organically grown produce (preferably from a small grower who you know is using natural composting methods and working to restore the integrity of the soil.)[2]

Secondly, avoid highly processed, denatured 'food products' and those substances which are known to take minerals out of the body, such as sugar and drugs (prescribed or 'recreational'.)[3]

Thirdly, reclaim some of the most mineral-rich foods known to humanity: sea vegetables. What? Eat seaweed? Yep. People everywhere across the planet have valued sea vegetables for countless millennia for their high mineral content. Here in Britain, we have always used a variety of them: purple-red dulse in Scotland and Ireland, samphire in East Anglia, dried kelp in every location (sea vegetables store well when dried.) Liverpool was originally called Laverpool because of the highly-valued green-black laver gathered along the northwest coast.

It's only in the past 70 years or so that these traditional foods have become neglected with the increase in factory processed 'convenience' foods. When you start using sea vegetables regularly in your diet,

---

[1] *"Lacking vitamins, the system can make some use of minerals, but lacking minerals, vitamins are useless" DOCUMENT 264, U.S.Senate, 1936.*
[2] *See 'Buy Old Food'*
[3] *See 'Beat the Sugar Blues'*

you will notice within a few weeks how the quality of your hair, skin and nails improves. Other commonly experienced benefits are smoother bowel function and improvement in problems of the female reproductive system.

Finally, in our quest for lost minerals, comes news of one of the most significant developments in the past 100 years: colloidal minerals. Created originally to address this modern problem of demineralisation, this natural product is made from minerals extracted from deposits of humic shale, created many millions of years ago from rotting trees and plants. These minerals, processed to a molecular size which makes them 98% absorbable by the human body, are then suspended in a liquid medium so all you need do is drink a couple of small capfuls a day to get a much needed mineral boost.

While I've never been keen on supplements of any kind (knowing them to be notoriously difficult to absorb), colloidal minerals are highly effective and making a real difference to people with busy lives.

Drink more rocks!

For further information re minerals, contact the information line number at the end of this book.

BUY OLD FOOD

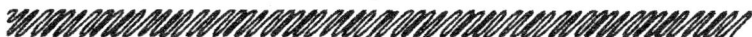

Think about it:

- you eat in a way that human beings never have before: chemically altered, highly processed foods, out of season, imported from climates very different from ours, unnaturally high in fats, added sugars and flavourings

- you eat foods that cannot sustain human health: mineral deficient, denatured, highly processed foods, designed to be 'mouth entertainment' rather than having any nutritional value

- you eat foods which directly create serious degenerative illness: even fairly conservative bodies like the World Health Organization recognise that the modern diet, high in saturated fats, refined flour, sugar and other 'empty' food products are responsible for the huge rise in degenerative conditions such as cancer, heart disease, arthritis, AIDS, M.E. and other immune system disorders.

While most people think this makes sense, the biggest obstacle to changing the situation is doctors. A G.P. friend (yes, I do have some) told me that, in all her years of training, she was offered only one day on nutrition - optional! You'd be as well off talking to a bus conductor about food and health as to a doctor. Time and again, clients inform me that their doctor has told them that food makes no difference to your health. So, the substances which we put into our body every single day, which are used by the body to build, repair and renew itself, cell by cell, have no connection to health! It doesn't matter, apparently, whether we create ourselves from plastic margarine and Big Macs or a wide range of nutritionally rich fresh foods - the results will be the same in the end. I'll leave you to decide on that one.

For those of us without the benefits of the latest medical training (and only common sense to work with), we have to turn to the wisdom about food handed down, generation to generation, for thousands of years.

Wherever we look, in cultures across the planet, the foods used to sustain human health were remarkably similar. By the way, I don't subscribe to the view of our ancestors as poor, wretched creatures, scrabbling to make a pitiful living and dying in misery at 35. These people had terrific health and strength (otherwise our species would have died out long ago.) It is we who have been abusing this constitutional strength and it is we who need to take responsibility and turn the situation around for the sake of future generations. There are still at least 18 traditional cultures on this planet whose people routinely live to 100-plus in good health, free of degenerative disease.

Here's the Traditional Foods Model:

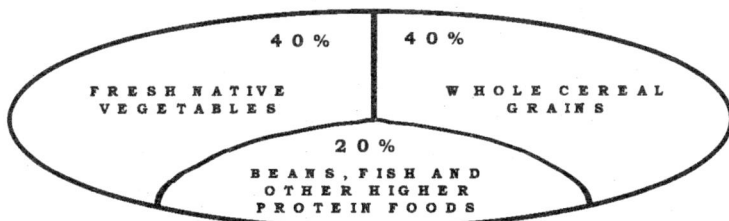

40 %
FRESH NATIVE
VEGETABLES

40 %
WHOLE CEREAL
GRAINS

20 %
BEANS, FISH AND
OTHER HIGHER
PROTEIN FOODS

The staple foods everywhere were whole cereal grains (e.g. whole rice, barley, millet, wheat, corn, buckwheat, rye etc.) Only recently have we tried to replace these staples with large proportions of meat, potatoes and refined flour - and we're paying the price with our health.

A huge range of fresh local vegetables accompanied the staple grains; for example, in Britain:

GREEN LEAFY VEGETABLES
such as kale, parsley, spring cabbage, watercress

ROUND VEGETABLES
such as peas, cauliflower, onion, pumpkin

ROOT VEGETABLES
such as carrots, radish, parsnips, turnips

Protein came chiefly from pulses (e.g. beans, lentils, split peas etc.) and fish. Meat and dairy foods played a much smaller part than they do in modern diet, being regarded as occasional delicacies (see 'Don't be a Silly Moo'.)

In addition to these basics was a whole range of supplementary foods:

sea vegetables
natural condiments
pickled vegetables
natural seasonings
beverages
native fruits, seeds & nuts
natural sweeteners

23

desserts and snacks

These foods produced a hugely varied cuisine (we live with the illusion of variety today; around 1900 for example, there were 10,000 varieties of apple in Europe - how many can you buy today?)

Only when we reclaim this heritage of nutritionally rich natural foods will we be able to step away from sickness and pitiful dependency on overworked doctors and the products of the pharmaceutical industry.

It's absurd yet true to say that most common ailments (recurring headaches, stomach upsets, diarrhoea, constipation, poor sleep etc.) clear up in a few weeks of beginning a grain and vegetable-based diet. Even more serious conditions benefit but you would be well advised to work closely with an appropriately trained healthcare professional.

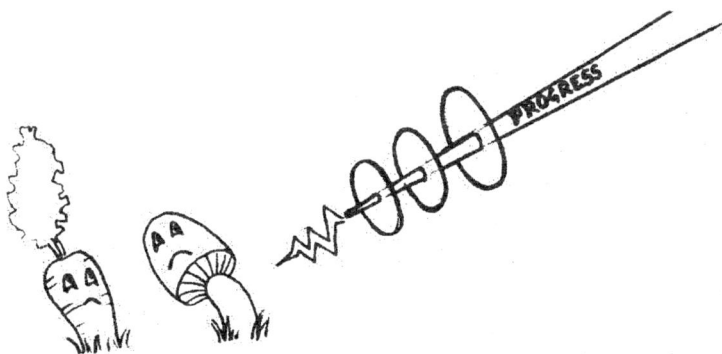

I urge you to rediscover these traditional foods. Please feel free to contact the information line number at the end of this book for suppliers, cookbooks, etc.

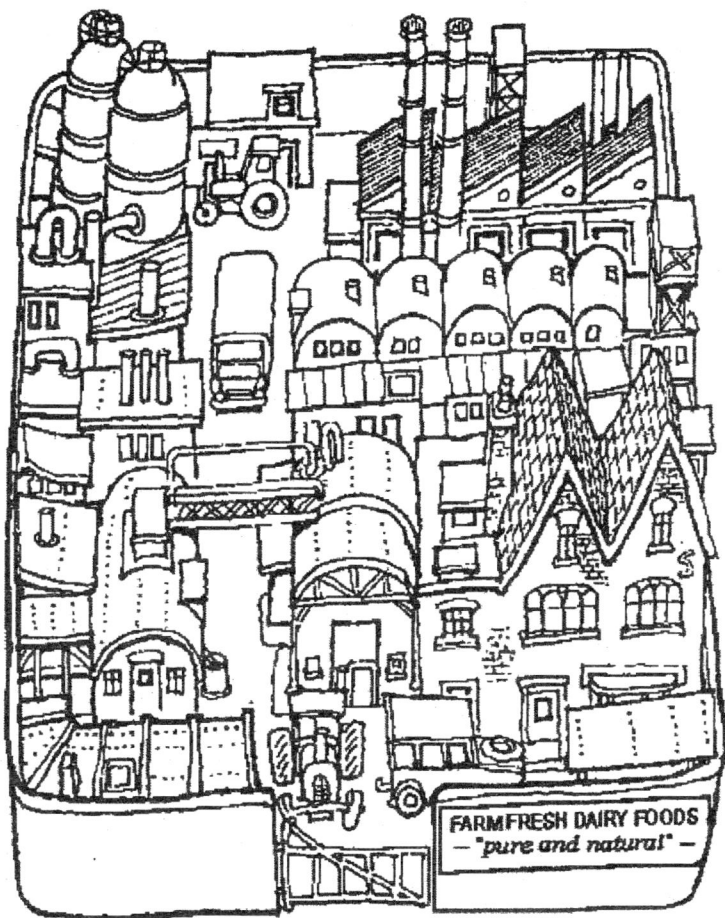

FARM FRESH DAIRY FOODS
— "pure and natural" —

BEAT THE SUGAR BLUES

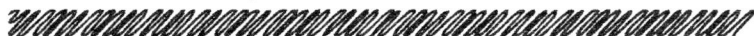

This is a subject which could easily turn into an entire book by itself, so I'll be as concise as possible.

If there is such a thing as karma, then sugar has a bad one. Next time you go to admire the pictures in Mr. Tate's fancy gallery in London, bear in mind that it only exists because of the 10,000 black bodies thrown overboard from the slave ships and the millions more rotting in the earth around the sugar plantations.

From the point of view of the health of those who eat it, sugar is a strong contender for the title of Public Enemy Number One

Let's look at just three of its effects:

- **Sugar robs the body of minerals. Everyone knows that it eats holes in your teeth; do you think that effect is magically contained to your mouth?**

Because it has no minerals of its own, sugar takes minerals from you for the digestive process. This, of course, links it immediately with a host of health problems, particularly those affecting the bones, e.g. osteoporosis, arthritis, rheumatism, osteomyelitis etc., but sugar is also heavily implicated in many psychological and nervous system disorders.

- **Sugar interferes with the body's natural blood sugar levels.**

When you take some sugar, it enters the bloodstream very quickly and raises the blood sugar dramatically. The pancreas (the organ in your body which regulates the blood sugar levels) starts pumping insulin like crazy to lower the blood sugar. When the effect of the sugar high wears off (pretty quickly), the natural blood sugar level is left lower than normal (this is why you can feel 'low' or depressed after eating sugar.) People don't notice this effect because they keep taking sugar to artificially boost blood sugar levels. Chronic conditions can result from this sugar-fuelled white-knuckle ride, the most common being hypoglycaemia or chronic low blood sugar. It's been estimated that 70% of people in the west are hypoglycaemic, the classic symptoms being spells of low energy and drowsiness. You can see it mid-afternoon in factories and offices across the nation as people's energy drops and they go off in search of coffee, tea, doughnuts, cake, biscuits etc., filled with the urgent need to raise their depressed blood sugar levels.

- **Sugar is addictive.**

If you don't believe this, stop sugar completely and see how you feel. Don't add it to anything and don't buy anything containing sugar (this is a challenge in itself, sugar is everywhere: soups, sausages, 'pure' fruit juices[1].) I've seen grown men weep for sugar as they tried to 'cold turkey' themselves off it.

The comment a few years ago by a Bristol University professor that sugar is "a drug masquerading as a food" is quite accurate. If sugar appeared today as a new

---

[1] *If a product contains 15% or less added sugar, it doesn't have to be declared on the packaging.*

product, it would be banned because its effect on human health is too strong.[2]

It doesn't matter what form sugar takes: white, brown, muscovado, demerara, molasses - the effect in the body is largely the same. Have you seen those little packets marked 'Raw Cane Sugar' in the cafés? What a triumph of marketing, to get away with calling refined sugar granules 'Raw Cane Sugar'! Perhaps if we re-name heroin 'Pure Poppy Extract' we can feel better about that, too. Honey behaves the same as sugar in the body; although it has been used throughout history, its use has been mainly medicinal, not added by the pound to make other things sweet.

When sugar first appeared in the west, it was kept in sealed jars on apothecaries' shelves because its effect was known to be so strong. The Elizabethans consumed about 2 lbs of sugar per head per year; today we consume 3 lbs of sugar per head per week!

If you decide to 'just say no' to the sugar pushers, simply replace refined sugar with more traditional sweeteners such as:

malted grain syrups (rice, barley, wheat, corn etc.)

natural fruit juice concentrates (apple, pear etc.[3])

pure maple syrup (go easy - this is the strongest natural sweetener.)

---

[2] *Artificial sweeteners, by the way, are no answer, being linked to problems such as cancer and liver damage.*
[3] *Don't give children blackcurrant juice to drink. No matter how natural it may be, it is strongly acidic and will rot their teeth.*

natural sugar-free jams

These will provide all the sweetness you need with none of the disastrous effects of refined sugar.

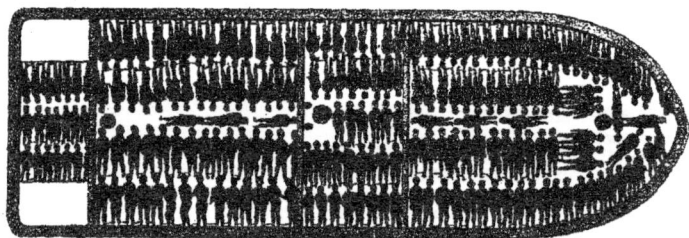

HMS FREE ENTERPRISE

DON'T BE A SILLY MOO

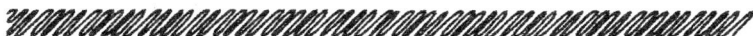

DRINKA PINTA MILKA DAY
MILK FOR HEALTHY TEETH AND BONES
MILK DOES A BODY GOOD

Did you, like me, grow up with this kind of stuff all over the place? Time to disperse a few more illusions.

Modern dairy foods are a nightmare. The meat and dairy industry uses numerous animal feed additives including antibiotics, tranquillisers, pesticides, drugs (the conditions the animals are kept in make them sick with infections such as mastitis), waste products (e.g. cement dust - USA; human excrement - France) and, in your favourite American burger, growth hormones. There is little concern or legislation governing the residues of these substances which find their way into meat and dairy products. Residues of antibiotics, for example, survive pasteurisation, which is only designed to kill off bacteria. (By the way, I've been told that calves fed pasteurised milk die within 60 days. The 'benefits' of pasteurisation are simply that dairy products last longer in storage and on the supermarket shelves.)

Even if dairy foods are 'naturally' produced, they are fundamentally unsuitable for human health. The 'calcium rich' image of dairy foods is a dangerous and irresponsible lie, perpetrated by the producers and marketers of the stuff. Dairy foods are highest of all in protein, and high consumption of animal proteins causes high levels of calcium to be excreted from the body - the exact reverse of the 'dairy foods for healthy teeth and bones' propaganda.

China, a nation which has never developed the use of dairy foods, has no osteoporosis and extremely low incidence of arthritis. The average American consumes 375 pounds of dairy products each year. The U.S. now boasts the highest incidence of bone fractures and osteoporosis in the world. The advice doctors give to osteoporosis and arthritis sufferers to "eat plenty of dairy foods to keep up your calcium" is like trying to put out a fire with buckets of petrol.

We are the only species on the planet that attempts to live on the baby food of another species - it's crazy. You wouldn't dream of leaping over a hedge, climbing underneath a cow and stuffing its teat into your mouth. Yet, if the mass producers put the greasy white fluid into bottles or cartons, people are happy to suckle on it. (This is why dairy foods are so addictive - "a nice milky drink helps you relax at night" - it's like going back to the teat to comfort yourself.)

Cow's milk, not surprisingly, contains the correct genetic programme to grow a cow. It is high in the proteins and minerals necessary to quickly create a huge, thick bone structure (the calf has to be up on its feet almost immediately after birth and grows its skeleton as fast as possible.) Cow's milk, however, is hugely deficient in the essential fatty acids necessary for neurological development (hence the low bovine presence on 'Mastermind'.) Moral: if your aim is to grow tall stupid adults, keep feeding the kids the greasy white stuff.

MORE PUS, VICAR?

Most humans lose the ability to break down and digest milk products by the age of three. After that, they just become problematic, indigestible sludge in the system - this is why dairy foods have the reputation of being the most mucus-forming substances on the planet.

There is a history of dairy foods. Roquefort, for example, the French sheep's cheese, was sold at the Roman markets. However, it differed in three major ways from modern dairy:

1. It was a 'live', unpasteurised product which contained enzymes that helped in its digestion (pasteurised cheese is essentially dead fat)

2. It contained none of the drug and other additive residues we discussed earlier

3. It was regarded as a delicacy, something which you ate and enjoyed occasionally as a treat (the Roman legions did not tramp along with Tupperware sandwich boxes stuffed with Roquefort butties.)

High consumption of processed milk products is another fashion we've been pressured into in order to line the pockets of big business: which do you think they care most about, your health or their profits?

Come on,

DON'T BE A SILLY MOO!

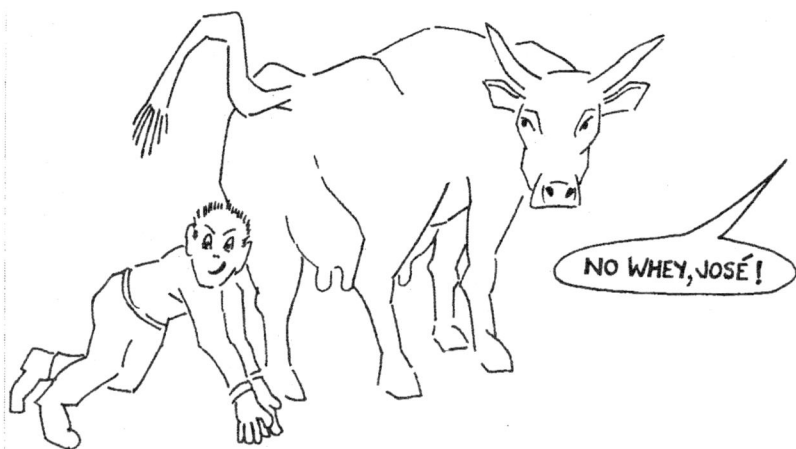

GET OFF THE BREADLINE

What is bread? Nobody knows any more. It's certainly not the stuff you buy from supermarkets and bakers today. Since the Industrial Revolution (and this has been the story with many other issues we've looked at in this book), the quality of bread and the ingredients from which it is made have degenerated alarmingly with disturbing consequences for human health.

So what has happened to our bread to cause such concern?

THE FLOUR USED IS BAD

Eighteenth-century aristocrats began the fashion for 'refined' flour, stripped of its nutritional value, which resulted in the chemicalised, sadly depleted white product most of us are familiar with today. However, any flour is rancid from oxidation eighteen hours after it has been milled, even from the whole grain. This rancidity is a major problem for health and is a factor behind the epidemic levels of allergic reaction to baked flour products in the modern world[1].

The best scenario is to make your own natural-rise bread, using a domestic-scale grain mill to make fresh flour. It may take a little longer than pulling the old "white death" off the supermarket shelf, but the illusion of "time-saving convenience foods" really comes home

---

[1] *Preservatives in the flour are, of course, only added with the aim of increasing the shelf life of the product. Their effect on health? Representatives of the funeral industry report that bodies now last longer without embalming because of the amount of preservatives they contain.*

when you lose months or years (or life itself) from
dealing with serious degenerative illness.

YEAST CAUSES HEALTH PROBLEMS

It was only at the beginning of the 20th century that
yeasts were added to bread (the idea came from French
chemists working in the wine industry.) As ever, the
reason for this was profit: to increase speed of
production. Yeast in the diet is linked to stomach
bloating, indigestion and weakened intestines. Also,
yeast increases the kind of candida yeast overgrowth
symptoms which are present in many degenerative
illnesses.

MODERN BREAD IS NOT BAKED

Commercial bakeries use something called the
Chorleywood Process (named after the place where it
was developed.) Dough is risen very quickly, using fast-
acting yeasts. It then passes through large rooms (you
couldn't really call them ovens anymore) where the
dough is blasted with hot steam to quick-
cook/pasteurise it, then passes by large heaters which
brown the outside. The whole process takes a fraction of
proper baking time. You know it's not properly cooked
because, when you take modern 'bread' out of its
wrapper and squeeze it in your fist, you've got dough
again.

Originally, bread was made using the natural-rise or
sourdough method, whereby the dough was allowed to
rise slowly in a warm place over a longer period of time,
during which it would take in natural yeasts from the
air. The bread was then thoroughly baked.

In the old days, the baked loaves were sometimes

hung on a rope to age. This naturally-fermented bread kept all year round without going mouldy. Whenever any was needed, a loaf was taken down, soaked in water, then re-baked, emerging from the oven just as moist and delicious as when it was first baked. This was strong, nutritious food and a couple of slices with soups and vegetable dishes made a satisfying meal (unlike the commercial 'edible cling film' which passes for bread today and which you can eat continuously without feeling satisfied.)

WHEAT IS NOT WHEAT

The grain used to make flour today is very different from that used in the past. Modern hybridised wheat, developed to produce higher yields at the expense of its taste and nutritional value, is linked with a host of health problems from weight gain to celiac disease. People with adverse reactions to wheat often find that they can tolerate two older forms of the grain:

SPELT - known for at least 9000 years, spelt has a delicious and hearty nut-like flavour. Back in the 12th century, it was praised by St. Hildegard of Bingen, who described spelt as the grain best tolerated by the human body.

KAMUT (pronounced "kuh moot") - this grain flourished in Egypt more than 5000 years ago. It contains gluten (like all wheat) yet most people with gluten-sensitivity can eat it without adverse effects. Its berry is more than twice the size of modern wheat and its light, delicate flavour is also surprisingly rich and substantial.

DEVITALISED FOOD DEVITALISES YOU

Modern bread and other processed flour products, because of their denatured and rancid state, form mucus in the body and, particularly in the digestive tract, sludge which clogs the system and prevents healthy digestive functioning.

While there may be a delicious smell wafting from the modern 'baker's shop', it's all achieved at a high cost to our health. Do a little research and discover what natural bread really is.

"GIVE US THIS DAY THY DAILY CHORLEYWOOD PROCESS"

(doesn't have quite the same ring to it, does it?)

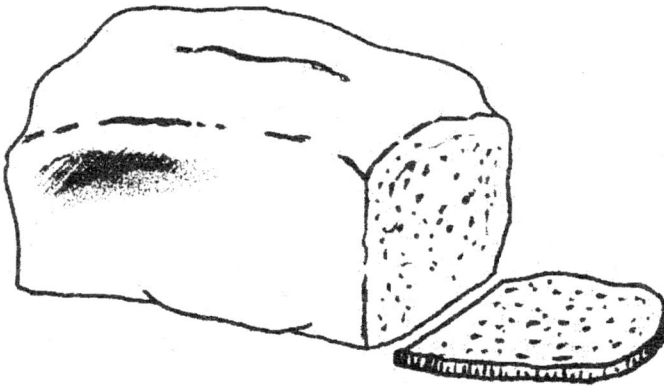

R.I.P.

DON'T GET A RAW DEAL

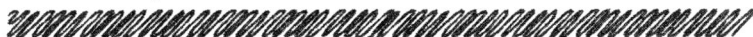

I wish I'd got a pound, as they say, for every young woman who has come to me for advice suffering from a familiar list of symptoms: pale, underweight, cold, with extremely low energy. They'd all been following 'healthy diets' from glossy magazines, usually promoted by Hollywood celebrities (you know, the 'Stella Spandex 480-day pineapple and prune diet for increased energy and multiple orgasms' kind of thing.) These diets all propound the illusion that healthy means raw.

The thinking with these régimes goes like this:

Raw food is pure and unadulterated and contains more nutrition than cooked food (which is 'killed' by the cooking). So, raw food is healthier for you.

Let's take a look at this.

- Raw food may contain all the nutrition but is that nutrition available to you? Raw food is actually the hardest to digest and assimilate, as you have to do all the work of breaking it down. Human beings invented cooking in order to begin the process of breaking down the food and making its nutrients available for the body.

- Eating a lot of raw food (and this is particularly true of tropical fruit and vegetables) cools the body. This is why we feel naturally drawn towards salads in summer - the cooling effect balances the warmer environmental conditions. In the same way, we want more warming foods (porridge, stews, hearty soups etc.) to balance the colder temperatures through the winter months. This natural order of eating appropriately with the seasons was the one and only option for our ancestors (pre refrigeration, chemical preservatives, motorised transport etc.) and is still the only option for those 18 or so traditional cultures still in existence whose people routinely live to 100 years and beyond in excellent health.

Today, in the developed world, we can completely upset the applecart. You can wake up on a freezing cold February morning and eat ice cream for breakfast; you can eat grilled meat all through a hot summer. Technology has allowed us to have access to anything and everything, and so we can do crazy things that go against the natural order.

Stella Spandex can get away with doing her wheat grass and beansprouts in the Californian sunshine but it's going to be a different story in Scunthorpe.

The buzzword in nutrition circles over the past three decades has been detoxification, the idea of 'cleansing' the body of impurities by consuming raw fruit, vegetables, juices and copious amounts of water. While this is a somewhat crude concept (the idea, for example, that large quantities of water will 'flush out' the kidneys like some kind of sewage pipe is a mistake - the kidneys are delicate filters which can become overburdened by having to deal with excessive quantities of liquid) there is nothing particularly wrong in principle with the idea of a short detox programme. The problems arise with the practical application of this stuff: basically, if you're in good health and in possession of a strong constitution, you may well benefit from the odd cleansing programme.

However, if you're ill, weak or unusually tired, you may do more harm than good by following an elimination diet; in this case, warming, strengthening foods may be a more effective route to recovery.

Generally speaking, a surer bet is to follow the Traditional Foods Model which we looked at earlier (see 'Buy Old Food'.) Whole grains, indigenous vegetables and fruits, fish, beans and pulses, sea vegetables, seeds and nuts will provide us with the most effective and practical quality and variety of nutrition we need to sustain good health.

Some raw food can be a useful addition to commonsense dietary practice (more in summer, less in winter) but bear in mind that hardy traditional peoples don't try to live on mango smoothies and wheatgrass juice, and neither should you.

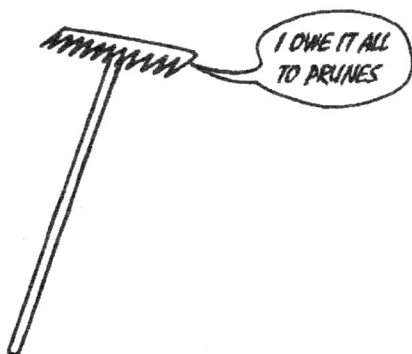

41

BANISH THE BELLADONNA

It is said that the indigenous peoples of South America, with revenge in mind for the atrocities they had suffered at the hands of the European 'explorers', made presents of seed potatoes to the white men in the full knowledge that, if the Europeans cultivated and ate them, the potatoes would rot their brains.

If this story is true, it certainly explains a lot about many of the issues discussed in this book!

True or not, the potato, member of the Solanum (nightshade) family, along with tomatoes and aubergines, is a strange food to have such a prominent place in our culture.

The Incas ate potatoes but took great care in their preparation. The potatoes (which were tiny compared to the modern version) were first immersed in running water for a long time, then dried in the sun (sometimes freeze-dried in the mountains). They were then ground to a powder which was only then used in cooking. In other words, the Indians knew the toxic properties of the potato and how to neutralise them. Today, we drop them into hot oil for a few minutes or zap them in the microwave!

Much has been said about the effects of potatoes, linking them with kidney stones, calcium depletion, physical and mental weakness, poor circulation and premature ageing. Two effects which clients have repeatedly reported to me are the connection between

43

potatoes and (a) poor quality sleep and (b) increased arthritic pain. Many, many times, clients have taken potatoes out of their diet and noticed an improvement in both of these areas.

It is a similar story with tomatoes. The Peruvian Indians gathered tomatoes wild (they were yellow in colour and the size of cherries) and made no attempts to cultivate them.

Again, clients report to me their own experience of improvements to health conditions, such as arthritis and skin diseases, when they avoid tomatoes.

For those in good health, treat them for what they are: an exotic delicacy to enjoy from time to time, but one which no sensible person would attempt to use as a staple food[1].

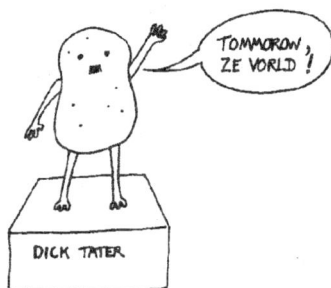

---

[1] *Potatoes, those huge swollen, watery tubers, are the second largest cash crop in the USA, after hybridised wheat. (Actually, they are third - marijuana is unofficially number one.)*

MEDICINE

SACK THE QUACK

For many years, they ruled the earth. Huge, lumbering creatures in positions of such dominance that they went unchallenged by the other life-forms on the planet, stamping on any opposition and growing fat on the back of others' pain and misery.

Are we talking Allosaurus here? No, just old sawbones.

GPs have had it all their own way for long enough. In a short space of time they have degenerated from being guardians of common sense and wisdom in the community to shiny-suited sales reps for the pharmaceutical giants. It is time they were replaced by something that works. Too harsh a judgement you reckon? Let's take a quick look at their performance...

Doctors are eager to stick labels on you: if you're feeling down, you're labelled 'depressive' and given addictive happy pills; if you've got aches and pains, you're given the label 'arthritis' and given powerful anti-inflammatory drugs (which can have disastrous side effects); if you are discharging excess gunk from your system through a skin rash, you get the label 'eczema' and are given hydrocortisone cream to send the discharge back inside again[1].

If you go with a headache to a doctor or pharmacist

---

1 *Hydrocortisone has side effects ranging from raised blood pressure to death. Every drug on the planet has side effects (often serious ones) - there are no exceptions*

they'll give you painkillers to take the pain away, completely ignoring the cause. If you get a cold, it's labelled an 'infection' and you're given antibiotics which will seriously weaken your immune system (so that, further down the road, you can pick up some other labels like M.E. or Aids.)

While there are keen and dedicated people in the medical profession, limited time and drug-biased training mean that the contribution of many doctors is reduced to scribbling on the prescription pad.

IT ISN'T FUNNY ANYMORE.

I know I promised no statistics but I can't resist quoting a few in this chapter (particularly as they come from the medical establishment itself, anyway.) Try this one:

PARACETAMOL KILLS MORE PEOPLE THAN HEROIN	
figures for 1998, deaths related to use of:	
ECSTASY	11
COCAINE	38
HEROIN	255
PARACETAMOL	561
Source: BBC RADIO 4 NEWS	

We could go on and on with this kind of thing but I think you're getting the picture. This stupidity has to stop. As I write, a friend who has decided to put her faith in doctors has been prescribed dexamethasone, a steroid. When I looked up the special precautions for this drug, they included "reacts with anti-epilepsy drugs" (which she is taking daily) and "do not use if you have cancer" (she has.) So many personal experiences like this are relayed to me, they just begin to look like the norm. Cancer is treated with drugs that cause cancer; a large proportion of the hospital population is there as a direct result of previous treatment.

Doctors receive virtually no training in nutrition yet set themselves up to guide us on health without this most basic understanding of the substances with which we create ourselves, cell by cell, day by day. We need to create a new breed of healthcare professionals who understand such basics as diet, nutrition, exercise, the importance of toxin-free household and personal care products, remedial massage and other natural treatments, and, finally, place emphasis on preventing illness rather than making fat profits for the drug companies from treating the symptoms of it.

CUT TO THE CHASE
Of course, one of the main functions of GPs is to refer you on to specialists and surgeons at the hospitals. Then you're really in trouble. Statistics time again:

UNITED STATES IATROGENIC (TREATMENT-CAUSED) DEATHS PER YEAR	
UNNECESSARY SURGERY	12,000
MEDICATION ERRORS IN HOSPITALS	7,000
MISCELLANEOUS ERRORS IN HOSPITALS	20,000
INFECTIONS IN HOSPITALS	80,000
NON-ERROR, NEGATIVE EFFECTS OF DRUGS	106,000
TOTAL	*225,000*
SOURCE: JOURNAL OF THE AMERICAN MEDICAL ASSOCIATION, JULY 2000	

This American death-rate represents at least 30 times the number of men and women who died annually during the Vietnam War. Millions protested against that conflict but the streets are strangely empty of outraged citizens screaming against this mass slaughter today.

The black humour in the above statistics lies in the fact that when the medical establishment gets it wrong (medication and miscellaneous errors) they kill 27,000 people; however, when they get it right by administering the correct medication (negative effects of drugs), they kill 106,000!

The figures for the UK are proportionately the same, being 40,000 deaths a year.

Have you ever wondered if there will be a World War III? It's happening right now and the phenomenal death toll (millions worldwide) is rising every year.

"Most cancer patients in this country die of chemotherapy" - Dr Allen Levin

Until doctors shake off the stranglehold of the pharmaceutical giants and evolve towards more effective practice, seeking clean and simple answers and preaching prevention before cure, then the only sensible and responsible guidance anyone can offer must be:

AVOID DOCTORS LIKE THE PLAGUE

For centuries, doctors have taken the Hippocratic Oath:

FIRST DO NO HARM

Let's harness all that hard work and dedication in the service of safe, effective healthcare which harms neither people nor the planet. Let's empower both the giver and receiver of healthcare to create for everyone the legacy of lasting good health.

We all know the argument: "If I was in a terrible car smash, I'd be so grateful to the surgeons for their skills in putting me back together". Well OK, but the vast majority of health problems are not like this and are perfectly preventable. We simply have to ensure:

- GOOD QUALITY FOOD

- GOOD NUTRITIONAL SUPPORT

- TOXIN-FREE ENVIRONMENT

- CLEAN WATER

51

- HEALTHY EXERCISE

- SENSE OF CONNECTION (TO NATURE/SPIRIT)

- PRACTICAL AND EFFECTIVE HEALTH ADVICE

The statistics alone show that the less you have to do with doctors, the longer you are likely to survive. If you decide to take responsibility for your health and future well-being, and you seek advice to help you on your way from any kind of healthcare professional, make sure that they address the seven points listed above. If they don't, get the hell out of there.

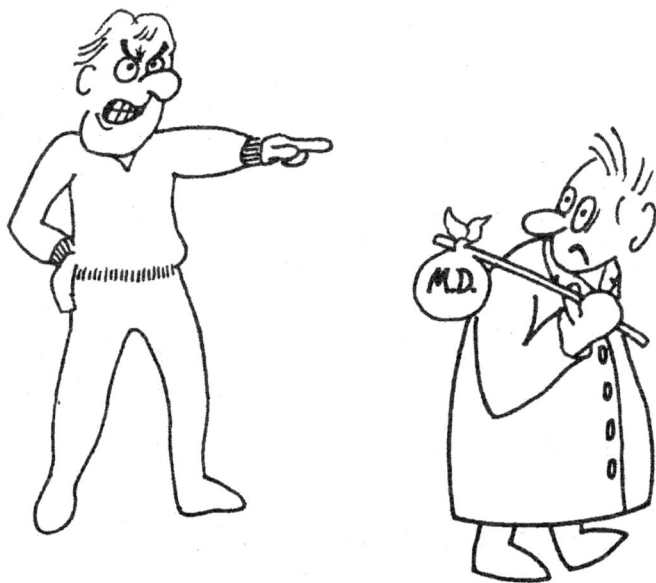

GET A LOUSY COLD

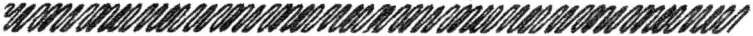

The concept of discharge in modern medicine is pretty well confined to the idea of waste material coming out of wounds and the natural orifices of the body during sickness. However, in traditional healthcare systems, discharge of excess material from the body was seen as a vital key to the maintenance of good health.

Here's how it works:

Every day, we take substances into our body's systems from the external environment: food, air, water and other liquids, and, if Russell Grant has got it right, subtle energies streaming in from the cosmos. Ideally, we should take in these substances, use from them what we need, then eject the waste material from this process through the natural exits of the body in the urine, faeces, sweat and exhalation. That's the ideal. What tends to happen in the modern world is that we take such quantities of material into our systems, or material of such poor quality, that our bodies are not properly nourished and we can no longer adequately discharge the excess.

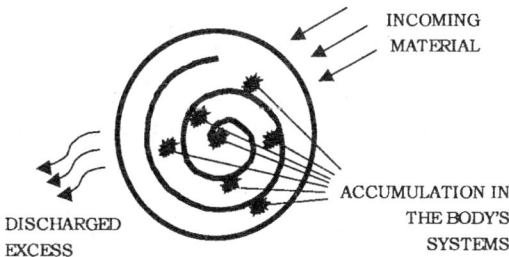

INCOMING MATERIAL

DISCHARGED EXCESS

ACCUMULATION IN THE BODY'S SYSTEMS

The result of this overload is that the excess which you simply cannot discharge accumulates in and around the major systems and organs of the body as fats, chemical residues and general sludge.

If this accumulation becomes too much for the normal discharge functions of the body, then the discharge becomes abnormal: skin rashes, eczema, so-called allergic reactions, conjunctivitis, asthma, headaches, diarrhoea, vomiting etc. etc.

There's an old saying: "If you keep doing what you're doing, you're going to keep getting what you're getting." If you do nothing to change this build-up of accumulation, it will eventually become too much even for the process of abnormal discharge, and then you're laying the foundations of serious degenerative illness.

In traditional oriental medicine, colds were seen as an important part of this discharge process. It was said that you should get a cold anything up to 4 or 5 times a year, usually as the seasons change over, to discharge any excess from the previous season. Like measles (which modern medicine would like to eradicate), like the tonsils and appendix (which western doctors consider expendable), colds were seen as an important part of the body's self-healing mechanism. Yet this, too, is seen by modern medicine as another enemy to combat and, ultimately, annihilate. Ask not whether nature has the wisdom to provide us with the simple means to cleanse and rebalance our systems, just pour those billions of pounds into subjugating something which will not bend to our brutal will.

But take heed, as an old teacher of mine used to say:

"If they ever find a cure for the common cold, God help us all."

CURE FOR LIFE FOUND
FROM OUR SCIENCE CORRESPONDENT

Scientists in Cambridge are thought to be very close to finding a cure for LIFE. This affliction, thought to affect most of the world's population, has so far baffled medical minds with its dangerous and chaotic complexity.

Considered by many to be a viral disease, probably transmitted by sexual contact, LIFE has up to now evaded all efforts by medical and pharmaceutical science to control its virulent and unpredictable growth patterns.

This latest breakthrough from the Cambridge team, led by Professor Ed Case, involves a straightforward medical procedure, elegant in its simplicity, visionary in concept.

Step 1 : the patient's brain (considered as the most likely site of infection) is surgically removed, then immersed in a cocktail of chemotherapy drugs to kill most of the cellular activity. The brain can then be safely returned to the cranium in its new state of toxified dormancy.

Step 2 : a simple computer socket is fitted to the back of the patient's head. This allows any type of computer terminal to be connected and input fed directly to the newly-receptive brain.

Praise for this ground-breaking treatment is already flooding in. Dee Monic, MD of the giant CONEM supermarket chain, comments: "Amazing! Tattooing barcodes onto consumers' arms will become a thing of the past, as will gruelling physical tasks like lifting supermarket loyalty cards. We are truly entering the age of the switched-on consumer."

Brave New World, indeed.

55

DODGE THE JAB

"There has never been any impartial and empirical evidence that demonstrates even remotely that immunisation does any good whatsoever."
PHILLIP DAY, INVESTIGATIVE REPORTER

"Now that there is a vaccine against it, measles has, by a strange coincidence, stopped being an annoying childhood disease and has, instead, become a deadly killer...
...Governments are either unbelievably stupid or else they are deliberately lying to help boost drug company profits."
DR. VERNON COLEMAN

"The British drugs industry is one of the finest examples of a technological industry... I am saying to the Government: please understand that if you continue to make an adverse environment for pharmaceutical companies ... they will start to move elsewhere."
SIR RICHARD SYKES,
CHAIRMAN OF GLAXO WELLCOME

The pressure on parents to have their children vaccinated is enormous. In the USA, children receive around thirty vaccinations by the time they go to school. There is a planned genetically engineered vaccine which will 'protect' against forty different diseases.

Current figures are impossible to obtain but here's a pattern from the 19th century described by Dr. Joyce Marshall: "In England and Wales, free vaccination was provided for smallpox in 1840, made compulsory in

57

1853, and in 1867 orders were given to prosecute evaders, therefore, few escaped vaccination."

Deaths from smallpox in England and Wales were recorded at:

1857 – 59 :	14,244
1863 – 65 :	20,059
1870 – 72 :	44,840

Dr. Marshall adds: "Deaths per year from cancer in England and Wales between 1857-72 also began rapidly to increase."

Beyond the bacterial and viral components of vaccines, there is a mind-boggling range of vaccine fillers, including:

aluminium

animal tissues (pig blood, horse blood, rabbit brain, kidneys)

formaldehyde (a neurotoxin)

glycerol (a component of antifreeze)

human aborted foetal tissue

monosodium glutamate

phenol (a disinfectant dye)

thimerosal (a mercury derivative)

As a vaccine researcher recently stated: "Would you mix this and feed it to your child from a bottle? Yet the government requires it to be injected with a syringe directly into our children's bodies."

If you have children and feel the need for support (and you probably will), seek out your local anti-immunization group. You won't have to go far to find one, they are usually formed by parents whose children have been affected by vaccination. In recent years, the number of adverse reactions to the MMR vaccine against measles, mumps and rubella has produced an increase in the number of support groups. The medical/drugs industry won't admit the possibility of a connection. The parents of children affected have, unfortunately, experienced the connection for themselves.

A final quote, simple and refreshingly candid from American doctor Joseph Mercola:

"Children do NOT get sick and die from some bad, scary virus unless they have some predisposing factors. The major ones would be eating sugar and drinking soda (fizzy drinks) and juice instead of water. "

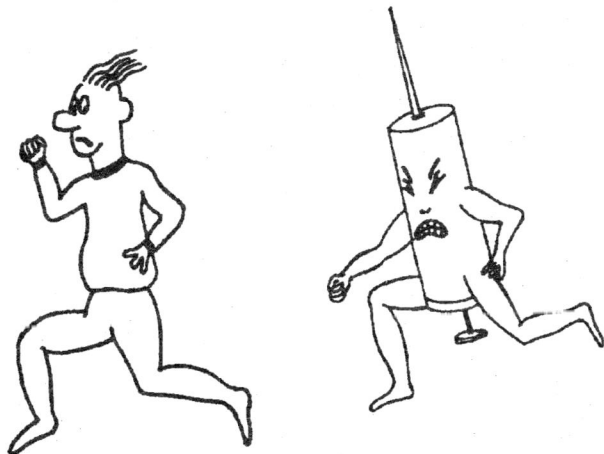

BE YOUR OWN DOCTOR

The vast majority of common ailments you can clear up yourself (or, at most, with the help of a friend or partner.) Get a good book on home remedies, keep some common ingredients in your kitchen, and you'll be prepared to deal with many simple health problems without wasting your time hanging around a doctor's surgery.

The approach is always the same:
1. Address the cause of the problem
2. Use an appropriate home remedy

Here's a handful of examples:

EARACHE

This problem affects children particularly (especially if they've had a lot of ice cream, cold juice and dairy products.) Without addressing the cause, this can go on to be labelled 'Glue Ear' by western doctors and, before you know it, your child is going through the trauma of having grommets implanted.

Clean up the diet, use natural sweeteners and seasonal fruits rather than junk, and only give cold things when the weather is hot.

For symptomatic relief, use a SALT PACK:

- Dry-roast one pound of natural sea salt in an iron or steel frying pan until it is very hot

- Wrap the salt in a cotton towel and tie up to make a flattened-ball shape

61

- Hold the salt pack against the ear (you may need to use an extra towel if the salt feels very hot against the skin)

- Reheat the salt when it cools, and re-apply the pack until relief is obtained

This remedy can also be used to ease stiff muscles and is effective on the abdominal area in the case of diarrhoea, menstrual or intestinal cramps.

CHESTY COUGH WITH MUCOUS

Eliminate dairy and other fatty foods from the diet.

To loosen mucous accumulation in the lungs, use MUSTARD PLASTER:

- Put two towels to warm on a hot radiator

- Add a little boiling water to a handful of plain mustard powder and mix to a light paste

- Spread the paste onto one half of a triple layer of kitchen towel. Fold in half so the paste forms the middle of a 'sandwich'.

- Spread a hot towel on the recipient's chest, place the mixture in the paper towels on top of the towel and cover that with the second towel

- Leave until the heat starts to feel uncomfortable (usually 10-15 minutes). The skin will become red, which is normal.

NOTES: Do not apply directly to the skin as it will burn. For children, mix the mustard 50-50 with plain flour.

HEADACHES

At back of head or deep inside: reduce salty foods, baked foods and animal foods. Drink warm, fresh-pressed apple juice.

At front of head or on top: eliminate any sugary foods, chemicals, spicy foods and coffee. Sip a hot tea made from 1 teaspoon of shoyu[1] topped up with hot bancha[2] tea.

INSOMNIA

Avoid nightshade vegetables (see 'Banish the Belladonna') and don't eat anything closer than 2½ hours before bedtime. To promote good sleep, do the following footbath just before bedtime:

- Place a handful of natural sea salt in a bowl of hot water.

- Immerse feet ankle-high for 3-5 minutes.

HYPOGLYCEMIA

If you get low blood sugar symptoms (energy 'lows' during the day, particularly mid-afternoon), avoid chicken, eggs and cheese and use SWEET VEGETABLE TEA:

- Finely chop or grate equal amounts of onion, carrot, white cabbage and sweet winter pumpkin

- Add the vegetables to four times the volume of

---

[1] *natural soya sauce (avoid commercial, 'Chinese restaurant'-type soya sauces.)*
[2] *mineral-rich twig tea, available from wholefood stores*

boiling water. Boil 3 minutes then cover and
simmer for 20 minutes.

- Strain off the broth, discard the vegetables.

- Drink 1 teacup of warmed broth every day in the
  mid or late afternoon.

NOTES: After it's made, this tea will keep for another 2
days in the fridge. Just warm it through before drinking.
Take this tea regularly until your energy levels stabilize
(in conjunction with good diet, this should be around 1
to 3 months.)

If any symptoms persist without noticeable
improvement, consult an appropriate health
professional.

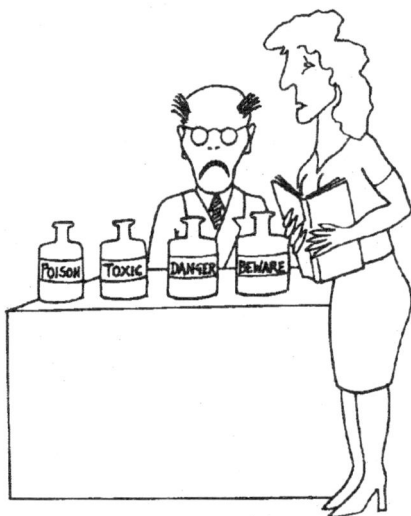

"I DON'T UNDERSTAND IT, DOCTOR. WE HAVEN'T
HAD A SINGLE CALL ALL THIS WEEK."

DON'T BE A WOMAN

If you want good quality healthcare from the medical profession, don't be a woman.

Womanhood has become a disease which you go to the doctor or hospital to be treated for. Let's take a look at some of the terrible ailments afflicting women for which they so desperately need medical intervention.

SEXUALITY

The assault on womanhood begins with the pill. The pharmaceutical giants promise unrestricted, unlimited, safe sex with no biological consequences (and, of course, no side effects - honest.) Aside from the many short-term side effects reported by women taking the pill, the longer-term effect of this horse-derived oestrogen product is to seriously upset the hormone balance within the body: the resulting condition, known as oestrogen dominance, is implicated in a host of health problems ranging from PMT to fibroids, osteoporosis to cancer.

PREGNANCY AND CHILDBIRTH

This is one of the biggest of all female health problems, involving continual medical tests throughout the pregnancy and a dash to the hospital so that doctors can remove the baby in a sterile, surgical procedure (the big fashion, at the time of writing, is for Caesarean section - brings the whole business much more in line with other surgical procedures). The baby emerges into a blinding-white, sterile, soulless environment, and then the tests and jabs can begin...

There is another way. So high is the probability of picking up an infection in modern hospitals, even doctors cannot argue against the fact that hospital is one of the least safe places to have your baby. If you are pregnant, find out about independent midwives in your area, particularly those who embrace more natural, traditional methods of childbirth. Unless you have a serious health condition which could affect you or your child, there is no reason why your baby can't be born at home (as babies always have!) and emerge in a beautiful, candle-lit, flower-filled room.

MENOPAUSE

When every aspect of a woman's biological cycles is regarded as a curse, then in step the drug companies and doctors to initiate curse management. When a woman enters menopause, her uterus and ovaries are shrivelled and useless, so just whip them out and put her on hormone replacement therapy for the rest of her life. Unfortunately, it's all based on an illusion.

Far from being "shrivelled and useless", her reproductive organs become active in new ways. The uterus, for example, becomes the main production centre for the hormone prostacyclin, which is believed to protect women from heart disease and blood disorders. All in all, a woman should be able to enter this new phase of her life intact, healthy and with fresh purpose.

The hormone balance in the body is disturbed by contraceptive drugs, HRT, oestrogens in the water supply and the food chain, and xeno-oestrogens (chemicals which mimic oestrogen) in the environment, from cling-film, plastic bottles, pesticides and fertilizers. The end result of this chemical onslaught is oestrogen dominance on a massive scale in the female population, linked, as we have already seen, with the epidemic levels of PMT, period pain, fibroids and other women's problems.

To address the problem of oestrogen dominance, the following steps are vital:

- eat organic-quality wholefoods (to avoid harmful residues, as much as possible)

- supplement with colloidal minerals

- avoid substances which disrupt hormonal levels [e.g. margarine, chemically processed cooking oils, soya, meat, dairy, drugs, plastics]

- replace sugar with natural sweeteners

- use a cream containing Wild Yam and Chaste Tree Berry [these herbs have been used traditionally for hormonal balance]

- use toxin-free toiletries, cosmetics and household cleaners

- do exercise that you truly enjoy ------- and be happy!

FOR MORE DETAILED ADVICE RE THE ABOVE ISSUES, CONTACT THE INFORMATION LINE NUMBER AT THE END OF THIS BOOK

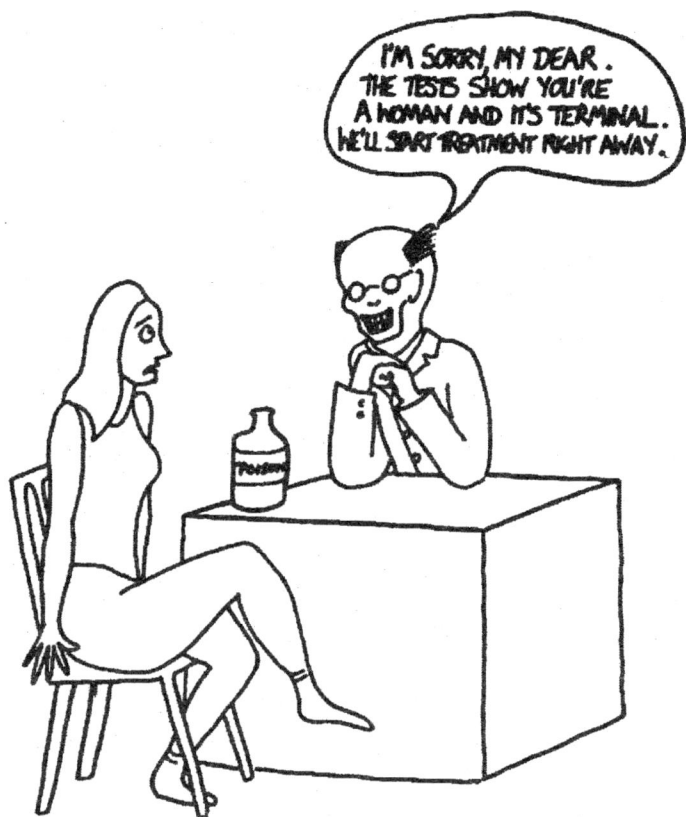

ENVIRONMENT AND CULTURE

HARD SELL, SOFT SELL - DON'T BUY IT

Let me start by offering you another little principle to guide you on your way through life's journey:

ANYTHING WHICH IS HEAVILY AND EXPENSIVELY ADVERTISED IS WORTHLESS IN TERMS OF ADDING TO THE REAL QUALITY OF YOUR LIFE.

When anything is heavily advertised, you should smell a rat:

- when you buy something which has been heavily advertised, you are paying for that advertising (which in some cases is more than the manufacturing costs of the product)

- only those products get advertised which create huge profits (you don't drive past billboards saying EAT ORGANIC CARROTS - although if governments had any concern for public health, maybe you should.)

Let's take one example. Some of the most heavily advertised products are cars. Sex, beautiful scenery, drama, humour, the thrill of speed, everything and anything is employed to persuade you to buy these damned polluting tin boxes. Fifty years ago, we could have had safe, clean-energy cars which lasted for

71

decades, but there's just not enough profit in that scenario compared to selling millions of petrol guzzling potency symbols with their ever-shorter 'planned obsolescence' lifespans[1].

So used have we become to operating our lives in response to advertising, the biggest multinationals have learned that, to ensure our 'brand loyalty', all they have to do is keep their logo in the public eye so that it becomes, quite literally, part of our environment: sky, trees, Mars, fields, houses, McDonalds.

Take a look at some of the advertising budgets allocated to ensure an endless supply of 'zombie consumers':

U.K. ADVERTISING BUDGETS - FIGURES FOR 1999	
MARS	£54m
COCA COLA	£44m
McDONALDS	£44m
ROWNTREES	£28m
Source: BBC, 'The Food Programme'	

All excellent nutritional material, of course.

---

[1] *Research reported by one of the motoring organisations showed that the most economical car in the world is the Rolls Royce. Such is the quality of the construction of the RR, it has a working life many times longer than your average loudly-advertised, quick-profit-generating tin box. In the same period of time, you'll spend more money repairing and replacing clapped-out motors than if you'd bought quality in the first place.*

72

Another aspect of the advertising onslaught is to simply make you feel inadequate or isolated unless you jump in and become part of the consumer feeding-frenzy. Youthful models with unblemished skin (computer-enhanced, in the pictures) are used to create images of 'perfection' which we are pressured to create in ourselves (with products which simply don't work - see 'Take Less Acid Baths'.)

There is enough stress and pressure in life without succumbing to this rubbish. Take the pressure off yourself: pursue true excellence and quality in your own life, on your own terms, and reject ridiculous illusions of perfection.

Oh, before we move on. The advertising budgets quoted above were quickly surpassed:

UK ADVERTISING BUDGET FOR LEAD-UP TO GENERAL ELECTION 2001	
LABOUR GOVERNMENT	£62m

What was that little principle, again?

ANYTHING WHICH IS HEAVILY AND EXPENSIVELY
ADVERTISED IS WORTHLESS IN TERMS OF ADDING
TO THE REAL QUALITY OF YOUR LIFE

Hmmm...

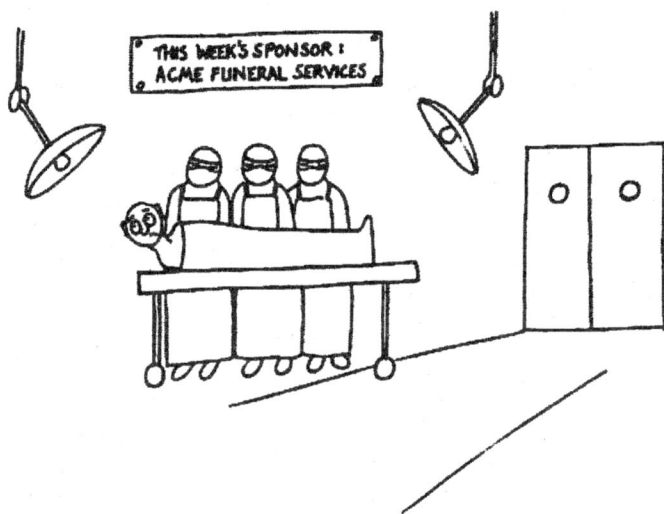

DON'T GET STABBED IN THE BACK

While many of the books on Feng Shui only succeed in making the spaciest new age groupie clench her buttocks in embarrassment, nevertheless the principles of this kind of traditional art (and all of the world's major cultures, it seems, possessed this wisdom) are grounded in common sense practices.

Good positioning in our living and working spaces makes sense however you look at it. Here's a simple guideline called The Power Position:

In any area where you regularly sit to relax or work, sit with your back protected by a solid wall, having a clear view of any doorway and, ideally, a pleasant view through a window.

The idea here is that no-one should be able to sneak up on you in a vulnerable position (the Chinese would say you could be stabbed in the back and, oddly, modern research seems to suggest that your stress levels are higher when you are in a vulnerable position such as having your back exposed to a door, window or other space behind you.) So, being able to see the door helps you to feel relaxed. Having a view helps in a similar way, too. Most of us feel better having some access to nature; the Chinese go further, saying if you have no view you have no future.

Don't simply accept this in some kind of superstitious way. Try it out. See if it makes a difference to your working position.

Here are some more basic principles:

- ensure no sharp edges or corners of walls or furniture point directly at you as you sit or work - they can make you feel tense and 'on edge'.

- choose pictures and decorative objects for their uplifting psychological effect - don't surround yourself with images of loneliness, anxiety, violence etc.

- when choosing a new home, ask what happened to the previous occupants - if there was ill-health, divorce, money problems etc., think twice.

- too much exposure to television, computers and other electronic equipment will make you weak - go out into nature to recharge your energy.

- if two or more children share a bedroom, place all the beds pointing in the same direction to lessen arguments.

- not making the progress in life you would like? Do a thorough 'spring clean' and clear out your clutter: old things which no longer serve you but which may have some emotional attachment which is holding you back.

GET TREVOR MCDONALD A PROPER JOB

I first sussed this one a few years ago, listening to a news bulletin on good old Radio 4. There was the usual list of disasters and atrocities then a final item tacked on the end:

"Four people were killed today when their car drove off the Tyne Bridge in Newcastle and plunged into the river below"

I pondered this for a moment, my enthusiasm for life lying in a defeated heap at my feet, then, suddenly, I got it! This item, like all the others, had been carefully selected. Why didn't the newsreader tell us about Betty Smith who died earlier that day after falling downstairs, or Jack Evans who died of a heart attack, or any one of the hundreds of people who died from all kinds of different causes that day? Why was that item selected over others? The answer is, of course, that it produces a thrill, an adrenaline rush of horror as we imagine the car plunging into the icy waters, the terrified occupants desperately clawing at the doors and windows as the car fills with water.

Apparently, dying in an horrific or unusual way makes you newsworthy; dying a more mundane death means you don't count.

It's sick. It gives an unbalanced view of daily life (how many people live in anxiety because of this stuff?) In addition, subjecting yourself to a daily diet of horror and misery is likely to result in feelings of helplessness (there is little we can do about most horrors and injustices) and numbness as we cut off in an attempt to survive this overwhelming emotional onslaught.[1] The detrimental effects of all this on our health and vitality can only be guessed at.

It makes sense to limit your exposure to this stuff and, when you do read, watch or listen, be aware that you are being presented with 'news' carefully selected for its shock value - you don't have to buy into it as a view of life. Give a tenner to help the flood victims, or whatever, but don't scare yourself to death!

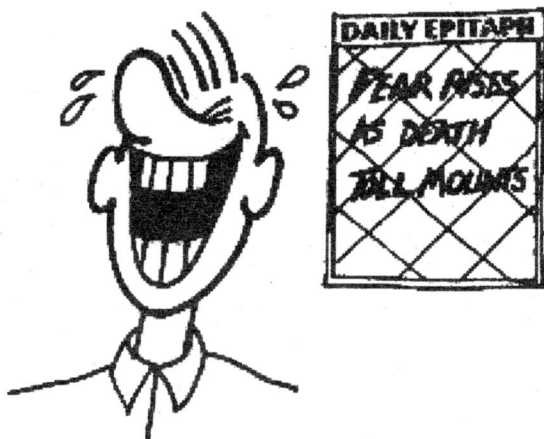

More insidious are the informative and 'good news' items. Often these are outright propaganda fed in the

---

[1] *On the other hand of course, genuine issues get short changed because of this voracious appetite for the next thrill. The genocide in Rwanda is one of the most appalling disasters of the last 100 years, yet once the shock-entertainment value had been milked, it disappeared from the news bulletins. The horror and hardship continue for these people.*

form of press releases from government departments and multinational corporations; you know the kind of thing:

"And finally, scientists in Cambridge are thought to be close to producing a drug which will eradicate breast cancer" (or heart disease, or aids, or arthritis etc.)

This is to let us know that those nice people in the pharmaceutical giants are making good use of all the billions of pounds from government, charities, jumble sales, sponsored walks etc., tirelessly working to create yet another miracle drug to benefit poor suffering humanity.

Well, don't buy it (literally). Their motivation is profit. If they were truly concerned with human health, they'd direct all that wealth and power towards commonsense health education and cleaning up the environment.[2]

By the way, don't hold your breath for a cancer cure. There never will be a pill you can pop to cure cancer because cancer isn't a disease in the simple sense (you don't catch cancer, for example.) Cancer is an overall degeneration of the body's major systems (immune, circulatory, endocrine etc.) To believe that one day we'll be able to clear up cancer with a little pill is a bit like saying we can save someone who is starving to death by giving them an after-dinner mint. It's hopelessly inadequate and looking in the wrong place.

---

[2] *But where's the profit in that. While I might make a quid from the sale of this book, offering you straightforward and effective advice, they can make hundreds of pounds from one course of treatment for one individual who then becomes dependent on their drugs for life.*

Finally, don't be fooled into thinking that you're getting more reliable information from the 'intellectual' newspapers than from the tit-and-bum tabloids. While the broadsheets may use longer words and employ more analysis, they emphasize the same issues as the gutter press, encouraging us to be interested in disaster, confrontation, misfortune and, nauseatingly, the comings and goings of politicians, aristocrats and 'celebrities'. Obviously, creatures such as you and I cannot match the importance of such godlike beings, floating from one glittering social occasion to the next, pausing only for the odd media interview to inform us of their brave struggle with a £1000-a day cocaine habit (or whatever).

Here's a little tip: next time you suffer a nasty attack of celebrity worship, just imagine your most awe-inspiring celebrity sat on the loo with their pants round their ankles, doing what we all have to do each day - works every time!

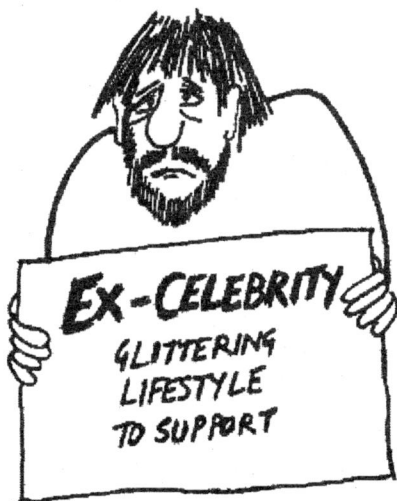

TAKE LESS ACID BATHS

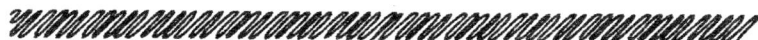

Here's a little story. There's no way to verify whether it's true or not because, if it is true, no-one in the position of being able to confirm it would come forward and do so. Anyway, see what you think.

Up until 1945, the outcome of the Second World War was uncertain. Every nation involved was developing, among other things, chemical weapons. In the west, the large chemical manufacturers were encouraged to develop and stockpile toxic substances for use in chemical warfare. The war ended, the chemical threat hadn't materialised, being overshadowed by the mushroom cloud of the H-bomb. The chemical giants were left with huge stocks of substances they no longer had any immediate plans for. What to do?

It was in the late '40s and '50s that we saw the huge explosion of cleaning products, toiletries, cosmetics and other 'personal care' products.

Take a look around a 'heritage museum' and see what was available before the last war: a few bars of soap, some soapflakes for washing clothes, a few brands of metal polish and wax polish, and not a great deal else. Today, there are more soaps than anyone could know about, vast quantities of shampoos, conditioners, shower gels, deodorants, antiperspirants, huge ranges of cosmetics, every kind of spray, bleach and cleaning liquid and scores of brands of 'air freshener' (which work not by freshening the air but by coating the inside of your nose with chemical fragrances.)

Endless supermarket aisles of substances which don't do what they say and are seriously damaging your health.

Here are just three very common substances and what I am legally allowed to say about them. Check the bottles in your bathroom and see if you can spot them:

ALCOHOL
A colourless, flammable liquid used frequently as a solvent and also found in medicines. It is believed that alcohol causes body tissues to be more vulnerable to carcinogens. Mouthwashes with an alcohol content over 25% have been implicated in mouth, tongue and throat cancers.

PROPYLENE GLYCOL
A form of mineral oil found in automatic brake and hydraulic fluid and industrial antifreeze. In skin and hair products, propylene glycol retains moisture content by effectively smothering the skin, preventing the escape of moisture but also hindering normal skin respiration by keeping oxygen out. Industrial safety data sheets warn users to avoid skin contact with propylene glycol as this strong skin irritant can cause liver abnormalities and kidney damage.

Propylene glycol is the main ingredient in baby wipes!

SODIUM LAURYL SULPHATE (SLS) AND SODIUM LAURETH SULPHATE (SLES)
These harsh detergents and wetting agents are used in garage floor cleaners, engine degreasers and auto cleaning products. Well-known as skin irritants, they are rapidly absorbed and retained in the eyes, brain,

heart and liver. Both SLS and SLES can react with other ingredients in shampoos and cleansers to cause potentially carcinogenic formations of nitrates and dioxins.[1] SLS is linked by many researchers with retarded eye development in children.

L'ORIBLE

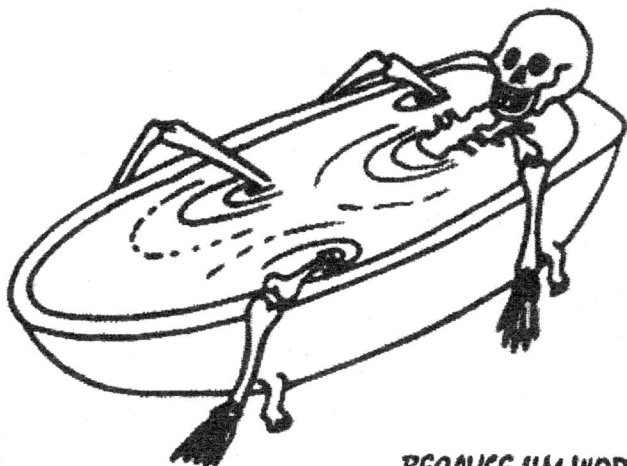

... *BECAUSE I'M WORTH IT*

One of the most amusing examples of cynical illusion perpetrated by the toiletries manufacturers is in shampoo. The vast majority of shampoos contain a significant amount of sodium chloride (salt to you and me). As you well know, you can dissolve a lot of salt in

---

[1] *DIOXIN was what the Americans called Agent Orange and was used to kill large areas of forest in Vietnam.*

liquid. This makes it a cheap bulking agent for shampoo manufacturers. You wash your hair with salt, what happens? It goes dry and stiff. So you feel the need to add conditioner to make it soft and manageable again. And who sells the conditioner? That's right, same people who sold you the shampoo. The conditioner 'works', often, because they don't add salt! (It's also more expensive than the shampoo of course.)

For information about ethical toiletries manufacturers, see the end of this book.

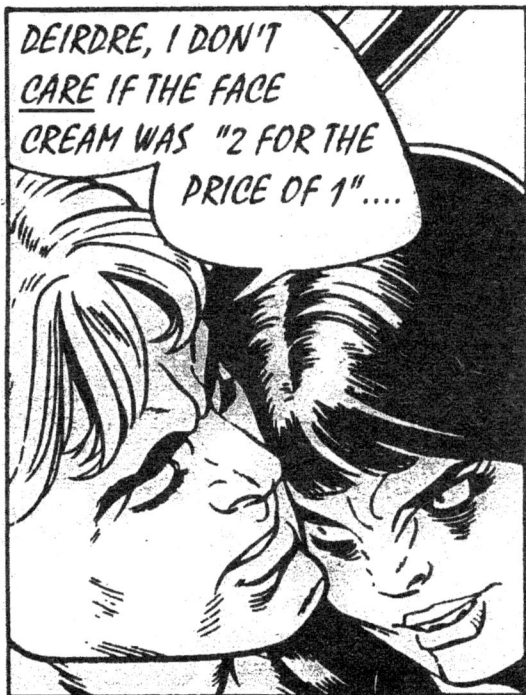

ASK YOUR GRANNY

The difficulty with offering people any kind of advice about health is that everybody thinks they've got it handled! Everybody thinks they eat well, take appropriate exercise and are aware of all the 'health' issues.

Traditionally, the skills for health and life were passed directly from mother to daughter, father to son. A few years ago, I met a man in his 70s who told me he could remember, as a small boy, going to visit his granny in Norfolk. She would always have a pot of stew on the stove and he noticed that she put a small strip of kelp seaweed into the pot at the start of cooking. She didn't know why (or she never said), but her mother had done it, and her mother before that. We can understand now that the kelp adds valuable minerals to the dish, but understanding of this kind has completely disappeared from most people's lives.

Here's a few tips your granny should have told you that could make a greater difference than you might think.

EXERCISE

While the fashion in 'healthy exercise' in recent years has been for punishing workouts with hi-tech equipment in gyms, unless you truly enjoy this kind of thing, DON'T DO IT! Pushing yourself to do things because you think you should is massively counterproductive! Punishing exercise régimes are like restrictive diets - you're likely to end up in some place opposite to where you thought you would be (slobbing out in front of 'Eastenders' with a box of chocolates, perhaps.)

The key to making anything work in life is to find the payoff, the enjoyment, the positive stimulus. Whatever works for you, be it walking down country lanes, doing housework, playing golf, leaping around like an idiot to heavy metal music - it doesn't matter, just go for what you find is fun and life-affirming, and do it on a regular basis.

COTTON
Wear pure cotton clothing, particularly next to your skin. Acupuncturists work very effectively by manipulating the flow of electromagnetic energy through and around the body (western science hardly acknowledges this energy, despite the fact that open-heart surgery is performed in China, the only anaesthetic being a few acupuncture needles.) This energy field is blocked by synthetic clothing (even wool, directly next to your skin, will block it.) So, wear undergarments of natural cotton (unbleached and organic, if possible - commercial cotton is one of the most heavily sprayed crops on the planet), and avoid synthetics (nylon, polyester, acrylic, polyurethane etc.)

COOKING
Cook with gas or other natural flame. The radiant rings of electric cookers generate a powerful electromagnetic field which zaps your e.m. field (in other words, your life energy.) Electric cooking also dries the food much more than gas so, if you're in a situation where you have to cook electric for a while, use more water in your cooking to compensate. If you live in a remote location where it's not possible to have piped gas, the camping-type cookers which use bottled gas are

surprisingly good - I've known several people get really good results with them.

Oh, and (as if I need to say it), AVOID MICROWAVES (see 'Modify Your Microwave'.)

NEW-FANGLED ELECTROCITY

My granny died a couple of years ago, aged 98, and she'd never used a telephone, declaring it to be "the Devil's work." While I wouldn't recommend going quite that far, it nevertheless makes a lot of sense to minimise your exposure to television, computers and other electronic equipment. In the case of T.V.:

- it generates e.m. radiation (about a metre deep all around the set - sit well back.)

- it replaces your active participation in life (watch 'Eastenders' and die - surely there's more to it than that?)

- the rapidly flickering images disturb the brain. Children, particularly, are affected by this: it can make them hyperactive the next day. Long-term, watching a lot of TV makes children lethargic.

- no-one truly understands the effect of continual exposure to horror and misery on 'news' programmes and depictions of violence in films and dramas - but I bet you could make a good guess.

If you work with computers, take regular breaks (the current E.C. guidelines are no longer than 20 minutes without a break) and keep plenty of healthy plants near the equipment to absorb e.m. radiation (it doesn't harm them, by the way!)

PLANTS AND AIR

Ensure there are soft-leafed green plants throughout your house, including the bedrooms. As we continue to decimate the planet of greenery, it becomes ever more important to fill our houses with healthy plants. They can absorb pollutants like e.m. radiation and carbon, and they recharge the atmosphere with oxygen and negative ions (when the ionic particles in the air are negatively charged, we feel bright, refreshed and awake.)

In addition, ventilate your home regularly, all year round, by opening doors and windows.

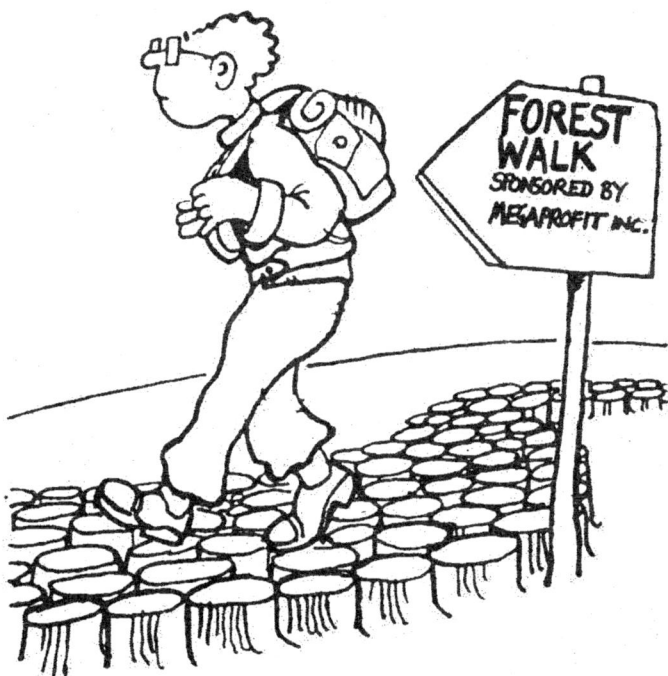

PYLONS

Don't live near electrical pylons. In the UK, around 500,000 people live less than 50 metres from power lines - 400 metres is considered to be the safe distance by scientists in the industry.

In the county where I live, North Yorkshire, the town of Northallerton has a great concentration of power lines; it also has an incidence of cancer well above the national average. Many researchers strongly suspect a link between those two facts.

There are an average 10-15,000 particles of pollution in every cubic centimetre of soil in the UK. These pollution particles become electrically charged by power lines and are thus able to stick much more readily to the lungs and other major organs. These deposited particles can then damage the internal organs and lead to cancer (particularly if the individual affected is deficient in minerals and other essential nutritional factors.)

DRINK SOLIDS, CHEW LIQUIDS

The same granny who never made it onto BT's Christmas card list, had another interesting characteristic: she always took a long time to eat her food. This made her the object of some gentle teasing at family gatherings but, on one occasion I decided to count: she chewed her food an average 40 times a mouthful. In many traditional cultures, this was seen to be essential practice for anyone wishing to enjoy a long, healthy and active life. It was said that solids should be chewed until they were liquid and only then could they be swallowed. Even liquids should be held in the mouth for a while, so they could mix thoroughly with the digestive enzymes in the saliva, rather than being gulped down. It certainly worked in my granny's case; she lived a long, active and hard working life, was an example to the rest of the family, and never seemed to lose her simple, generous, loving nature.

GO TO FRANCE TO EAT

Do you remember that fuss, a few years ago, about red wine and heart disease? Somebody had taken a look at the European table for deaths from heart disease and noticed that France, supposed home of heart-unfriendly rich cooking, was actually way down the list (about no. 14). We in the UK were, of course, in the top 3, with the town of Dewsbury given the accolade of 'Heart Disease Capital of Europe' - supposedly because the chip shops still used lard for frying!

Some bright spark asked: "What is the difference between us and France? Of course, they drink red wine!" So, research grants were handed over and the eggheads set to work, trying to isolate what chemical in the red wine prevented heart disease and make a drug from it. GIVE ME STRENGTH! None of these clever clogs thought to enquire as to what else the French might do. Let me offer a few points of enlightenment.

- the French regard eating as very important and they give it time: in towns across France, everything closes down at midday and the people spend 1½ to 2 hours enjoying (and digesting) their lunch in a relaxed way. (OK, I know it's probably different in Paris, but they've only got themselves to blame.) You certainly won't see anybody running down the street, mobile phone to one ear, stuffing a sausage roll into his mouth.

- in the evening, it's customary to eat *en famille*, enjoying the food with family and friends. Again, a sociable, unhurried, relaxed atmosphere.

- they eat fresh vegetables with their meals. The markets in the little towns display a wondrous variety of produce of which the French are understandably proud. Every small restaurant will serve good quality fresh vegetables which balance the fattier or higher-protein elements of the meal. (You'd be forgiven for thinking that the Brits' idea of a fresh vegetable is baked beans.)

Do you think these factors might just have a little influence on the picture, too?

Keep searching for those magic chemicals, boys.

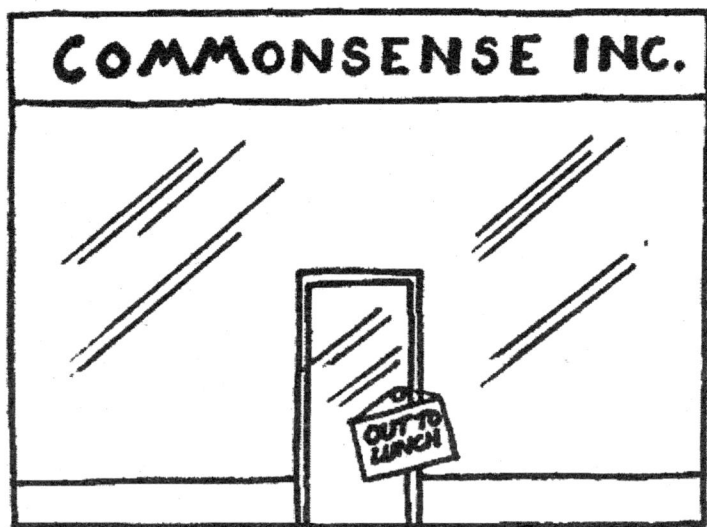

DON'T DRINK THE WATER

Remember that saying, 'Don't drink the water'? It used to refer to certain dodgy foreign countries where profit, corruption, apathy, vested interest, ignorance and other factors, all took precedence over considerations of health, resulting in (among other things) water unfit to drink.

Growing numbers of people are taking increasingly powerful medicinal drugs (antibiotics, steroids, hormones, sleeping pills, painkillers, tranquillisers etc. etc.) On any given day, **half of the population are taking a prescribed medicine**. This doesn't include all the non-prescription drugs bought over the counter at chemists and supermarkets. Many drugs are excreted in the urine after their initial effect on the body. Up to 75% of a dose of a tranquilliser may be excreted in the urine, other drugs may be as high as 90%.

Waste water is often discharged into freshwater rivers (this is the point at which we hear of researchers discovering that the fish near sewage outlets have changed sex.)

Drinking water supplies are often taken from these same rivers.

The purification technology employed by the water companies was designed many years ago - before doctors started prescribing such huge quantities of drugs for all these millions of patients, and before the problem of removing drug residues had even been thought of.

Let's ask some obvious questions:

- when you turn on the tap, are you getting a cocktail of analgesics, antibiotics, chemotherapy drugs, heart pills, hormones and others?

- is there a risk that water supplies will be so contaminated with drug residues that anyone using ordinary drinking water will be effectively taking drugs?

- if male fish in certain rivers are becoming female, could female hormone residues in the water supply affect the development of human babies[1]?

No one seems to know.

No one in authority seems to want to know.

Politicians on TV drink bottled water.

What does your common sense say?

---

[1] One American researcher has gone so far as to speculate whether the last baby boy has been born in the USA who will be able to reproduce by normal means.
Source: Dr. John Lee, "What your Doctor may not tell you about pre-menopause."

TOOTH DECAY – TRUTH DECAY → FLUORIDE
We can deal with this one quite simply:

- the term 'fluoride' covers a wide range of fluoride-based chemical additives which are put into the public water supply, toothpaste and foods. These fluoride compounds are in fact hazardous industrial waste [by products of the fertilizer and aluminium industries for example] which are used without detoxification procedures being carried out beforehand.

- all of the recent large-scale studies on fluoridation and tooth decay show that FLUORIDATION DOES NOT REDUCE TOOTH DECAY. However, what tests <u>have</u> shown is that from 8% to 51% of children drinking fluoridated water have dental fluorosis, the first visible sign of fluoride poisoning.

- independent research in Japan and the USA has linked fluoride compounds to various types of cancer.

"[Fluoride] is a toxic waste product of many types of industry; for instance, glass production, phosphate fertilizer production and many others. They would have no way to dispose of the tons of fluoride waste they produce unless they could find some use for it, so they made up this story about it being good for dental health. Then they can pass it through everyone's bodies and into the sewer."
Dr. John Lee, Marin County, California.

MODIFY YOUR MICROWAVE

Here's a nice little technology. Originally developed by the Nazis to eliminate the need to find cooking fuel during the invasion of the Soviet Union (they'd also, no doubt, got some other charming little applications in mind for microwave radiation.) The Soviets took a look at this technology after WWII and decided there were just too many hazards associated with it. They finally banned the use of microwave apparatus in 1976.

An American researcher in the late '70s produced a report on the harmful effects of microwave ovens. He mysteriously disappeared and it wasn't until the late 1990s that evidence of the dangers of microwaves was published. These dangers include:

- disturbance of the hormonal balance in the human body

- breakdown of the human electromagnetic energy field

- loss of memory

- loss of concentration

- increased percentage of cancer cells in the blood

In 1990, researchers in Berlin heated samples of water in a variety of ways then used the water to help germinate grain. Grain watered with the microwaved sample did not germinate.

Don't just accept this, though. If you're so inclined, test it all out for yourself.

Alternatively, you may want to follow the John Darrell Guidelines for Safe Use of Microwave Ovens:

- remove the plug from the socket

- with a pair of wirecutters, neatly snip off the plug from the mains lead

- cover the microwave oven with a cotton cloth (colour and pattern of your choice)

- place a healthy green plant on top

This novelty plant stand will be an attractive addition to any modern kitchen and, I guarantee, will make a positive contribution to your and your family's health.

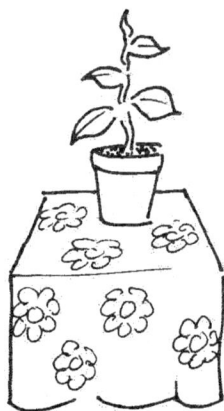

ESCAPE THE RAT RACE

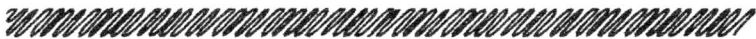

Oh, yes. We've all heard about them. Wicked, illegal pyramid schemes where people in the lower ranks are duped into working to line the pockets of those at the top with obscene profits.

Do you know which of those schemes is the most disgustingly exploitative?

A JOB

Think of your average big corporation. At the top, there may be one guy or, perhaps, a small group of directors / CEOs etc. After that, upper management: blue chip double-diamond starship commanders or whatever. Then middle management. Then lower management (office managers, tea bag vice-presidents etc.) Finally ... the cannon fodder.

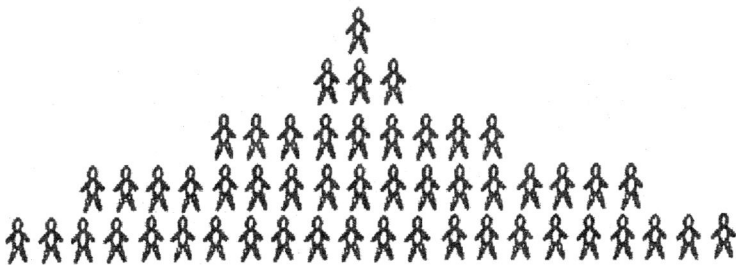

Now, if you're operating in the middle-ish part of the heap, you're probably having quite a tough time right now. You've heard all the gossip and seen all the stuff on TV and in the press, you know: "There's no such thing as job security anymore"; "Well, we were hoping to give a five per cent rise this year but, with the Chancellor's recent warnings about the downturn in the economy, it'll have to be two per cent" and so on and so on. So, you work hard all year, neglect your family, put your own development on the back burner, and the company does well. The guy at the top gets a £¼ million bonus and you get your two per cent (maybe).

This is a 40 to 45-year[1] pyramid scheme rip off that gives you a life of quiet desperation, a two-week package holiday each year, gnawing anxiety at your inability to get on top of the credit card bills and, waiting at the end, the golden reward of a state pension. (Although if you couldn't get along financially when you were working full time, quite how you're supposed to manage on a pension is anybody's guess.)

Better minds than mine have calculated that, at any one time, in free circulation in the world's economies, is enough money to make every man and woman on the planet wealthy.

Now don't get me wrong. I'm not trying to drag some half-baked notion of communism in through the back door here, but what is very clear is this: money is simply a form of nature's abundance like any other, and you can choose to work to direct it into someone else's pocket or you can make the decision that you have a worthwhile contribution to make in this life and can create the money to make your biggest dreams come true.

---

[1] *Assuming that you start work around the age of 20*

ESCAPE THE TRAP

The structure of business is changing — although relatively few people know it yet. The old system, developed during the Industrial Revolution, is now so unwieldy and inefficient it is collapsing — jobs lost by the tens of thousands, job security gone etc.

In the old model, goods are manufactured cheaply abroad, then importers bring them into the country (administrators, truckers etc. etc.), then packers are involved, printers, marketing companies, distributors (more wholesalers, administrators and truckers) and, finally, individual stores (in reality, it may not end there — entire businesses are formed around the stuff which the big stores no longer want, involving yet more administrators and truckers.) The whole system is so bloated and inefficient it is collapsing before our eyes, along with its army of parasites.

There is a natural evolution taking place away from this old model and towards a system with far greater integrity and sustainability. Whenever you have a good experience, there is something which you are likely to do: tell someone else about it. If you see a great film or go out for a wonderful meal, you'll tell your family, friends, acquaintances etc.

Network Marketing began in the USA about 25 years ago as a way of operating outside of the conventional system which was already groaning under the weight of 'middle men.' NM does away with the parasites. This frees up a huge amount of money (anything up to 85% of the cost of a product can be taken up by advertising and distribution). By 'conversationally marketing' this new approach to people, you benefit by receiving high commission rates (made possible by the money now available which previously went to the 'middle men') as the people you introduce order the products they want direct. There is no hype, deception or pressure at any stage — you are simply showing someone how to use a great new system.

Through NM, people can access the highest quality, most effective products[2] which, if they had to go through the old system, would become so expensive they would be beyond the reach of many.

The vision behind NM is of a fairer distribution of wealth. The money goes to those who are directly working to create it. Because of the nature of networking, as the people you've introduced introduce people themselves, you can quickly build a strong network which generates an excellent income for you (incomes several times those of standard jobs are commonplace in NM.) This is the direct opposite of the pyramid scheme because you only benefit by supporting the success of those you introduce. As they are more successful, so your income increases.

The benefits of NM include:

- be your own boss

- choose the hours you work

- create residual income with unlimited potential

---

[2] *e.g. nutritional products, toxin-free toiletries, cosmetics and other personal care products, household and automotive products etc. etc. (see TAKE LESS ACID BATHS)*

- develop a rewarding business by empowering others and developing new skills

The aim of this book is to point you away from restriction and limitation, and towards those things which really work. If NM is something you'd like to investigate further, contact the information line number at the end of this book.

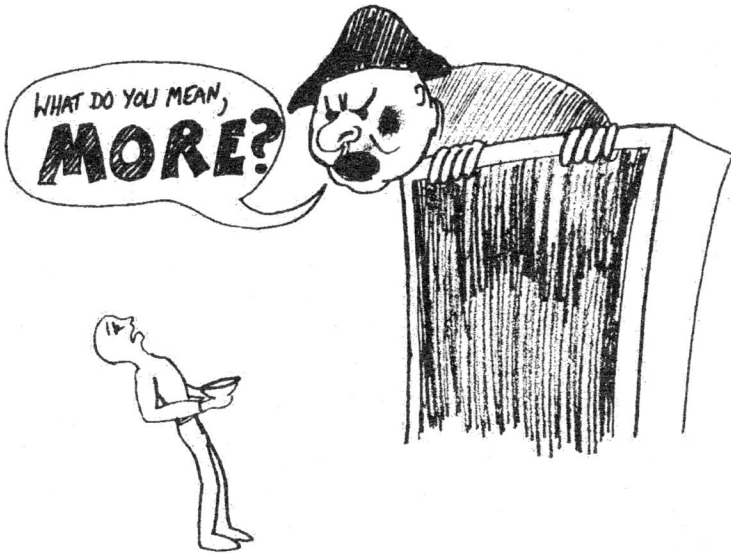

A FEW LITTLE SUGGESTIONS

get plastic out of your life

laugh

scrap sugar

delete dairy

get a cold

don't accept the norm in society

read more fairy stories

make real bread

use truly toxin-free personal care products

relax

drink clean water

enlighten and support your local community

minimise air travel

do exercise that you enjoy

don't vaccinate your children

be in charge of your own behaviour and life direction

learn wholefood cooking

enjoy great sex

don't vote, it only encourages them

chew well, swallow only liquids

keep life simple

eat food that feels good <u>after</u> you've eaten it

don't teach children, give them the right space to learn

if you can't read it, don't eat it

don't scare yourself to death

do work that doesn't damage people or the planet

get a compost bin

be your own doctor

drink more rocks

don't retire from something, retire to something

sack the quack

keep uplifting pictures in your home

eat when you're hungry, drink when you're thirsty

make friends and spend time with them

have self-respect rather than self-doubt

do well according to <u>your</u> standards

get a hobby

take responsibility for your life

leave everything better than you found it

INFORMATION LINE

///

For information on toxin-free personal care products and safe, effective nutritional supplements, phone the number below.

For further information about any of the issues raised in this book, how to source useful organisations, foods, books, etc., telephone or fax:

01751 – 472327

Would you like to be kept up-to-date about new titles from Regeneration Publishing and talks by John Darrell? Tell us your contact details and we'll send you the latest (and we <u>won't</u> give your details to junk mail companies.)

REGENERATION/JOHN DARRELL
SOUTH VIEW
AISLABY
PICKERING
YO18 8PE

01751 – 472327 (tel/fax)
Join our e-mailing list:
<u>john@regen2002.fsnet.co.uk</u>

LET'S TALK

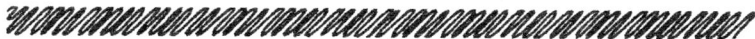

Do you belong to a club, society or other group who would like to hear John Darrell talk about creating health and happiness?

Would you like a personal lifestyle consultation with John? Contact us now on:

01751 – 472327

john@regen2002.fsnet.co.uk

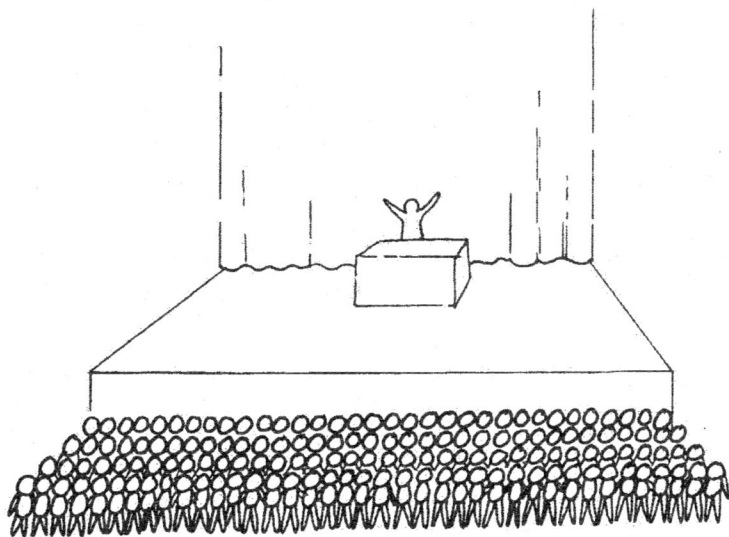

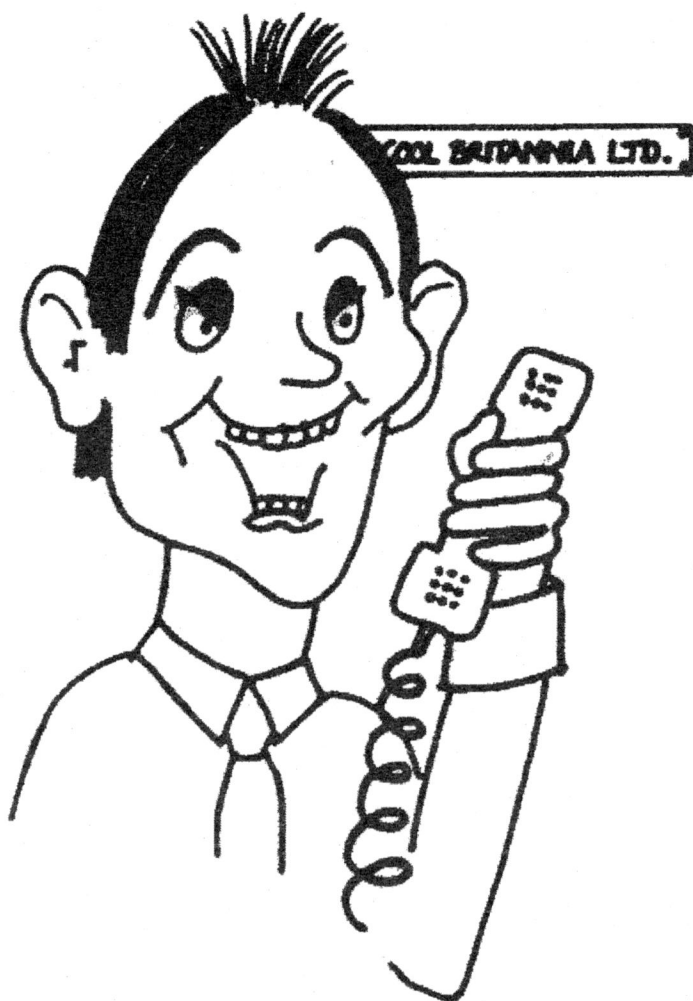

"Hi John, it's Tony. Send us 55 million copies, will you? Everybody in the country should read this!"

ORDER ! ORDER !

The information contained in this book is important. Much of it is difficult to find elsewhere, and it is often suppressed or ignored by those who stand to profit from the *status quo*. We are glad to have been able to make it accessible to you.

Continue this process of enlightenment and empowerment by sending copies to family, friends and open-minded acquaintances

EAT LESS PLASTIC, DRINK MORE ROCKS
£ 8.95 (INC. P&P)

REGENERATION PUBLISHING
ISBN   0 – 9543281 – 0 – 8

To order, contact 00 44 (0) 1751 472327 (tel/fax)

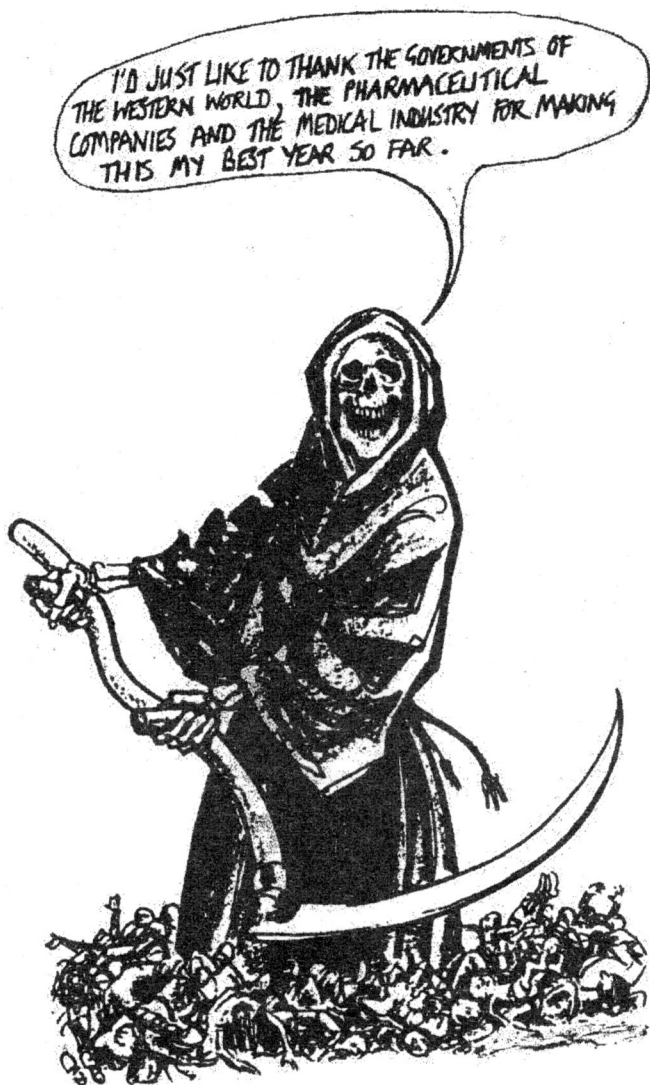

...AND DON'T FORGET:

vaccines are safe

beef is good to eat

chemotherapy cures cancer

supermarkets put your health first

advertisers and the media tell the truth

politicians work for the good of the people

genetic engineering will make the world a better place

... and beware of low-flying pigs!